Trust Me,
I'm (Still) a Doctor

D0587603

Also by Dr Phil Hammond

Medicine Balls
Why Does it Hurt When I Pee?

Trust Me,
I'm (Still) a Doctor

Dr Phil Hammond

BLACK & WHITE PUBLISHING

First published 2008
This updated edition first published 2009
by Black & White Publishing Ltd
29 Ocean Drive, Edinburgh EH6 6JL

1 3 5 7 9 10 8 6 4 2   09 10 11 12 13

ISBN 13:   978 1 84502 261 7

Typeset by RefineCatch Limited, Bungay, Suffolk
Printed and bound by CPI Cox & Wyman, Reading

In memory of Bob Sang, an inspirational leader
and my finest source ever

Thanks To

Jo, Will and Ellie
Miles Kington
Ian Hislop
Private Eye
Michael Mosley and the *Trust Me, I'm a Doctor* research team
The Observer
The Independent
Jan Poloniecki
Maria von Hildebrand
Ernest Codman
Heidi Beck
Alison Young
Andrew Foster
Black & White
and
all of my sources

CONTENTS

PREFACE TO THE SECOND EDITION

People behave differently when they know they're being observed. Ask your MP. Would you claim expenses for moat cleaning and mole catching as 'necessary to perform your parliamentary duties' if you knew they'd be published? Probably not. And neither would you tart up a string of second homes at public expense and trouser the profits tax-free. But what if you were told that these perks were the secret entitlements of an exclusive club, to make up for your disappointing salary? How many of us would be tempted to throw in such parliamentary essentials as a patio heater, a duck refuge and a luxurious wet room? Or bill the taxpayer for your daughter's rent or your boyfriend's dry rot? Fifty years on from *Animal Farm* and we're back where we started.

No profession — doctors, MPs, bankers, priests — can effectively regulate themselves in secret because professional and institutional loyalty masks the worst excesses of human behaviour. We need public scrutiny to ensure people in authority open ranks and use their power responsibly. The trick is to make that scrutiny as constructive as possible, so it encourages us to address our failings and helps us do a better job. In contrast, destructive scrutiny is obsessed with fear, blame and central control. If doctors and nurses spend all day chasing the wrong targets, you pretty soon lose sight of the patient.

In twenty years as an NHS whistle-blower, I've learnt that the feedback that can really make a difference to patient care comes from the front line, not from Whitehall. For every scandal I've exposed, the staff, patients and relatives knew something was badly wrong long before the various establishments saw fit to act. And when they did act, it was usually with the retrospective panic of knee-jerk over-regulation.

Since the Public Inquiry into the Bristol heart scandal a decade ago, we've had a Commission for Health Improvement, a Healthcare Commission, a Care Quality Commission, a National Patient Safety Agency, a Commission for Public and Patient Involvement, a National Institute for Health and Clinical Excellence, a Monitor for foundation hospitals, the revalidation and re-licencing and for doctors, the slavish promotion of patient 'choice' and a whole raft of quality, safety and access targets. And yet, still we have the corporate manslaughter of dozens of patients in Maidstone and Mid Staffordshire due to appalling standards of care.

The messages of this book are simple. The success of NHS depends on training and motivating staff, and giving them the time and resources to do their jobs properly. To help us, we need leaders brave enough to ignore all the extraneous bureacratic crap and focus on quality and safety. We need to collect and publish outcomes that matter to staff and patients. This includes listening to those on the receiving end of poor care or dangerous working conditions, and acting on what they say. Instead of isolated whistle-blowers being taken outside and shot, NHS workers and users should unite and speak up, so errors can be learned from and stopped, rather than repeated and hidden until the body count is too high to ignore. MPs and bankers may dabble with independent regulation of their behaviour, but what matters is the experiences and opinions of those people they serve. So it should be with the NHS.

INTRODUCTION
Unlucky Dip

'Knowledge is knowing that a tomato is a fruit.
Wisdom is knowing not to put one in a fruit salad.'

Miles Kington

It's 22 years since I qualified as a doctor, and I'm still amazed (and touched) that anyone should trust me. Most people would run a mile if someone ginger honed in on them with a cheesy come-hither grin (check the cover), but wearing a stethoscope somehow makes it alright. There are times when you have to trust a doctor, like when your blood pressure has fallen off the scale or there's a piece of bone sticking through your leg. But there are also times when it's worth asking the odd awkward question. Such as 'would you mind washing your hands first?', 'have you actually done this before?' or 'is this the best drug you've got, or merely the cheapest?'

Healthcare is a lucky dip. Our aim is to 'do the right thing right': spot the diagnosis quickly and give you the best available treatment with clean, steady hands and lashings of compassion. The reality is that medicine is complex and unpredictable, and there are lots of competing demands. Too many people get the wrong care – wrong diagnosis or treatment – or they get the right treatment wrongly given – delayed or bodged.

The NHS has traditionally blamed its shortcomings on a lack of funding. Not having enough doctors, nurses, cleaners, drugs, training, sleep and machines that go 'ping' adds up to a pretty dangerous mix. It's like climbing aboard a plane with a bit of wing missing, a hole in the fuselage and a pilot who's never flown before, who hasn't slept for 72 hours but is determined to 'have a go'. Miraculously, or rather because of the expertise and dedication of the staff, 90% of patients are 'satisfied' or 'very satisfied' with their NHS care. But it's not always a safe system to work or be ill in. 10% of patients and staff – often the unhappy ones – are damaged (physically and psychologically) by being in the NHS.

When I qualified in 1987, the 'training' mantra was 'see one, do one, teach one'. You'd see someone do a liver biopsy, either in the flesh or on *Casualty*, and off you'd pop with a large needle to have a go on some unwitting patient before teaching the next doctor how to do it. My first liver biopsy was a partial success with a very long needle – I got a bit of liver, a bit of spleen, a bit of kidney and a bit of bladder. More of a kebab, really. But the patient was effusively grateful: 'You've gotta learn somehow.'

There was so much dangerous dabbling, but no-one wanted to talk about it for fear of frightening patients. So I formed a double-act called *Struck Off and Die* with Tony Gardner and we tried it out about as far away from our workplace as we could find (the Edinburgh Fringe). It was more of a therapy session than a comedy, but it got us invited to a BBC Radio Light Entertainment Christmas party, where I followed the Beverley Sisters down the stairs and Ian Hislop into the toilet. I offered him a column for *Private Eye* and washed my hands afterwards.

I've been the *Eye*'s medical correspondent for 18 years, and I'd like to think I've been a fierce advocate for a safer and fairer NHS. Unfortunately, no-one takes much notice of angry exposure in a satirical magazine written under a pseudonym (MD). As I've got older, and closer to being a patient, I've tried to move away from just exposing bad healthcare to understanding it. But not excusing it. We're now putting over £100 billion a year into the NHS and we deserve a good service for that money.

The bulk of this book is the distilled wisdom of over 400 *Private Eye* columns, originally published as *Doing the Rounds* and, more recently, *Medicine Balls*. The book is helpfully divided into 'Blame the Tories' and 'Blame Labour'. I've name-checked health secretaries to fill us with nostalgia (or nausea). Health Secretary is seldom a good career move, and almost invariably ends in failure because you've stoked up expectations you can't hope to deliver in the time frame. So you panic and introduce wave upon wave of untested reforms that leave the staff giddy and bitter.

If the last 60 years have taught us anything about the NHS, it's that politicians shouldn't try to run it from Whitehall. Lord Darzi, ex Labour Health Minister and robot-assisted surgeon, at least tried to put doctors back in charge before resigning to spend more time with his robot.

So can doctors be trusted, once again, to run the NHS? Certainly more so than politicians. Especially if we work in teams with other professionals, accepting criticism and feedback from patients, and knowing the limits of our competence. In the last 20 years, I've exposed enough medical scandals to make your head explode. These aren't exclusively the fault of doctors, but just hammer home the point that doctors are human. We may be very bright and reasonably ethical, but if you put us in an unsafe, underfunded and unaccountable NHS and throw in a touch of arrogance and self-interest, it can pretty soon turn pear-shaped.

Doctors are their own harshest critics and many of the stories I've written about have come from whistle-blowing medics. I've also met those on the receiving end of medical accidents, which has stoked up my anger but also provided inspiration. Most don't want to blame and sue, but to understand what happened and prevent it happening to someone else.

The biggest scandal I've uncovered is the Bristol heart

disaster, but the NHS at that time was full of 'Bristols' – staff with inadequate resources and expertise getting bad results but struggling on regardless because there was no mechanism to help or stop them.

I hope the NHS is safer because of what happened in Bristol, but as only heart surgeons publish their results it's very hard to tell. A lot of our money now seems to go to shareholders, rather than safety. As the late Paul Foot put it: 'there has been an enormous transfer of power in Britain from public, elected authorities to private, unelected corporations.' And they don't invite scrutiny.

After the Bristol inquiry in 2001, Labour had a real opportunity to put quality and safety at the heart of the health service, but Tony Blair soon tired of that and decided instead to feed the NHS to the market. Unfair competition, commercial secrecy, duplication of services, distrust of management, job insecurity, intimidation, bullying and an obsession with profitability are not the ingredients of safe healthcare. Everyone who works in the Department of Health and the NHS should (re)read and digest the Bristol report. If they had, the recent tragedies in Maidstone and Mid Staffordshire could have been averted.

This is my contribution to the debate, charting my journey from lean, angry stand-up junior doctor to fat, angry sit-down GP. One of the delights (and embarrassments) of performing comedy is that you get immediate feedback, good or bad. But in medicine, outcomes are much harder to measure, and often we don't bother, so you could be a mass-murdering GP and still have a heaving (but slowly diminishing) waiting room.

The Tories and Labour are now falling over themselves to publish outcomes, such as talking to patients and finding out if they can still hop and skip a year after their hip replacement or heart surgery. 'Patient-reported outcomes' are becoming all the rage and require feedback from those on the receiving end. Early results suggest that we spend £144 million a year operating on people who had no significant complaints about their health beforehand or find that their condition is worse or no better afterwards.

In an ideal world, we'd assemble all these outcomes, adjust them for risk to make sure those treating sicker patients are fairly represented, and then compare one team's figures with the average of all the other teams' figures in the UK, for each procedure. If a unit fell below an agreed safety standard (e.g. double the average mortality or complication rate elsewhere), this would prompt a swift investigation (in a supportive, grown-up way) to find out why (and to protect patients).

Unfortunately, the Government and medical establishment aren't rushing to set standards, perhaps because they're worried they might be sued by those who don't reach them. So publication is going ahead and it's left to patients to decide their own standards. Do you want to go to hospital X, which is on your doorstep with cheap coffee and easy parking and a mortality rate for your operation of 16%? Or do you want to travel 50 miles to hospital Y, where you don't know anyone and you couldn't afford to park even if you could find a space, but the mortality rate is 4%? It's called 'patient choice'.

One of Labour's key reforms, 'Shifting the Balance of Power', is known in the Department of Health as 'Shifting the Blame onto Patients'. Now that patients have 'choice', they have to accept responsibility when things go wrong. I think this is cruel and not terribly wise, but that's politics for you. It's never been a tougher time to be a patient. So I've concluded this book with a 'Speak Up' guide for those outside the anaesthetic who want to ask the odd awkward question.

There's also a cut-out-and-keep membership card for the Royal College of Patients, for you to display prominently on your bedside locker or handbag. It's a virtual organisation that I've founded to take on the might of the medical establishment. Everyone is a vice president, whether you want to be one or not.

Gabby Logan is the Royal Patron. No matter how much money we put into the NHS, it will only get safer and better if patients find their voice: 'As Vice President of the Royal College of Patients, I was wondering how likely it is that you're going to kill me?' It might just make all the difference. Good luck, and let me know how it goes.

Dr Phil
August 2009
drphil@bbc.co.uk

BLAME THE TORIES
1988-1997

BLAME THE TORIES
1988-1997

I entered medical school in 1981, two years into Thatcher's first
term and a year after the Black Report which nailed home the
point that poor people get sick, and that the best way to
improve health is to conquer poverty. Thatcher promptly
buried it.

Norman Fowler was in charge of the Department of Health
and Social Security for all my student years (1981–87), and
somehow managed to prevent Thatcher from privatising the
NHS. In 1986, he launched a memorable 'AIDS: Don't Die Of
Ignorance' campaign (or 'ADIS: Don't Die Of Dyslexia', as the
posters were changed to). Despite a speech impediment, Fowler
gamely tried to lecture us on the importance of proper condom
usage, a message lost on Cecil Parkinson, and kicked off the
first in a long line of over-hyped health scares by stressing the
point that 'everyone is at risk' from HIV infection. Leaflets were
promptly dispatched to 23 million households, half of which
contained either an elderly couple or an old person living
alone. As one elderly, hypothermic Dorset woman commented
in the *Guardian* (January 15, 1987): 'Do you think this caring
government would swap my AIDS leaflet (as new) for a bucket
of coal?' Better still, pile them high and burn them to keep
warm.

The most profound change of the Fowler era completely
passed me by as a student. Thatcher invited Sainsbury's chief
Roy Griffiths to reform the NHS and he announced, in 1983,
that we needed general managers at every level of the service.
Anyone who couldn't get a job in a supermarket promptly

3

jumped ship to the NHS. The health service clearly needs excellent management, but the Tory appointees were a mixed bag intent on burying bad news and bad debt, and silencing dissenters. In such a climate, quality and safety could never flourish.

KENNETH CLARKE
July 1988–November 1990

Fat Ken became health secretary on the back of a funding crisis, but fought off Tory plans to scrap the NHS and replace it with an insurance-based system. Instead, he utilised his new army of managers to reform the service along business lines, arguing that an internal market would somehow improve productivity and reduce costs. The NHS was divided into 'purchasers' and 'providers', and money was supposed to follow the patient anywhere he or she wished to travel. Alas, block contracts soon stopped any freedom of movement. The purchasers ran out of money every winter and the providers stopped treating patients, unless they happened to be those of GP fundholders, who seemed to have more money than everyone else.

Clarke claims to have come up with the idea of fundholding on the back of an envelope whilst in the bath, relaxing in a gentleman's way (or something like that). He wound up some GPs by telling them: 'Every time I mention the word reform, you reach for your wallet,' and annoyed them further by suggesting what they should do with their time. But entrepreneurial GPs grasped the nettle, improved the care of their patients and pocketed the profits.

Clarke was an unrepentant beer-and-cigarillos jazz buff. His dedication to the nation's health was further questioned when he became deputy chairman of British American Tobacco and voted against the smoking ban. Fellow MP Alan Clark called him 'a puffball' and 'a pudgy life-insurance risk', but Clarke survived Clark. Managers loved him for leaving them alone to get on with commercialising healthcare. Lots of beans were counted and boxes ticked, but the NHS still seemed pretty dangerous to me.

Expenses Update

Ken Clarke managed to avoid paying the full rate of council tax, on either of his two homes, by effectively claiming that neither is his main residence. He has agreed to pay the full rate in future but defended his past behaviour.

THE INDEPENDENT
Fringe Medics Show Death Wish

10 August 1990   By Miles Kington

My Edinburgh withdrawal symptoms are quite severe this year. Having been involved in most of the last 15 fringes, I badly need that dose of adrenaline, camaraderie, excitement, dirty socks and staying up far too late for fear of missing something. Last year I was with *Instant Sunshine* at the Pleasance for two weeks. This year, nowhere.

What makes it worse is that for the last three months I have been getting posters and leaflets for Edinburgh Fringe shows through my letterbox. As, however, I am a hard-eyed monster of egoism, and jealous of anyone actually going there, I have remained totally unaffected by these Fringe hopefuls.

With one exception. Phil Hammond, a junior doctor from Bristol, is going up with a fellow doctor, Tony Gardner, to do two things of such extraordinary difficulty that even to attempt them smacks of a death wish. He clearly needs all the help he can get.

The first is to rescue the good name of medical humour. Every year, medical student groups go to Edinburgh with material that might provoke hoots of laughter at the hospital Christmas show, but is groaned off the stage in the real world.

Shows with names such as *Medicine Balls*, *The Enema Within* and *Just a Little Prick*.

Well, medics have to deal with the crude side of life, so their escape from it is equally crude. When you are the one made responsible for pain and misery, it is wonderful to be irresponsible for a while. Those doctors who rise above it into other levels of humour (J Miller, G Garden and R Buckman) have usually escaped from medicine as well.

The extraordinary thing in medical humour is that one target is never aimed at. The doctors themselves. The whole medical set-up. The whole crazy, overworked, underfunded, killingly tired, hierarchical, nepotistic health service is never got at. You can make jokes about bowels and rubber tubing, but never about drunken consultants or doctors getting a commission from cremation forms. Hammond and Gardner reckon they are the first doctors in the revue field to rise above lavatorial level and have a go at the way medicine is run in this country. Two, as I say, hard targets.

I know just how hard it is because when I first teamed up with *Instant Sunshine* twenty years ago, the other three were still junior doctors and absolutely terrified that playing with such a group would ruin their careers; afraid senior doctors would get the impression that they were not serious chaps. I was in charge of writing concert and programme notes, when needed. For 10 years they would not let me mention their medical connections, which, as they were (and are) full-time doctors left not a lot to talk about.

It was a ludicrous situation. It was ludicrous that when they went for job interviews, they were scared stiff that one of the panel might have seen them playing. It was ludicrous that junior doctors who were not even guilty of criticising the regime (they thought much of the system asinine, but went along with it in the same way as chaps at boarding school do) felt they had to behave as if they were.

'How do your doctors make time for *Instant Sunshine*?' people ask me.

'They let their patients die,' I tell them.

This is not true. It is junior doctors working for 80 hours non-stop who have to let their patients die. But Hammond is the first medic to get up on stage and get a laugh by saying so. There is a chance he might be putting his job on the line. In many medical contracts, there is an extraordinary clause forbidding doctors to talk to the Press. There is, as far as I know, no medical contract which says the doctor may not go to Edinburgh and there make fun of his employers on the stage, but there doesn't really need to be. Not in the medical profession.

I haven't met Hammond or seen the act, but I like the sound of someone who, because junior doctors get less than £2 an hour overtime, hands out badges to the audience that read 'I earn more than my doctor'. I like someone who says: 'The reason we draw the curtains when a patient dies is so the doctor can raid the fruit bowl without anyone seeing.' I'd like to think he sells out at Venue 6, Celtic Lodge, Brodie's Close, Lawnmarket, 12–25 August inclusive, from midnight to 1.15am. Good luck, lads.

Struck Off and Die
Programme Notes

August 1990

Struck Off and Die are two tired and surly junior doctors, Tony Gardner and Phil Hammond, who got together to publicise our working conditions and wage a war of ridicule on the medical establishment. We encourage criticism (and chocolates) and are especially keen to hear from anyone who has felt the rough end of the NHS pineapple (confidentiality assured, all letters answered, photo appreciated). Concessions for this show are available for NHS staff and the relatives of anyone we've killed. Sorry.

Some Facts
- Junior doctors work on average 90 hours per week (Dowie 1989).
- Every third week, most work a continuous 81-hour shift for which a house officer earns less than £2 an hour before tax.
- The CEPOD Report (1987) highlighted 140 preventable surgical deaths at the hands of overtired, unsupervised juniors. Ennis and Vincent (1990) found that human error and lack of supervision were at the heart of 64 obstetric disasters.
- Drug addiction rates amongst doctors are 30 times the national average and they are three times as likely to die of cirrhosis and four times as likely to commit suicide. No figures are available for church attendance.
- Less than 1% of consultant surgeons are women, and only 6% of physicians. It doesn't help if you're black, either.

Thought For The Day: Is killing patients when you're tired – and then killing yourself – the only way to learn?

WILLIAM WALDEGRAVE
November 1990–April 1992

William Waldegrave took over when John Major came to power, and told a reporter he'd 'rather be back in the Foreign Office.' Waldegrave never seemed comfortable as health secretary, nor with a commercialised NHS. As he put it: 'The NHS market isn't a market in the real sense . . . it's competition in the sense that there will be comparative information available.' Alas, the comparative information was largely about cost and productivity, and not anything that told patients about the quality and safety of their care.

Patients could still use the press to raise questions about the NHS, but Waldegrave wasn't too keen on that either. On March 23, 1992, in the run-up to the election, he sent a letter to the editors of regional newspapers: 'I write to urge immense caution in the use of individual case histories where the NHS is alleged to have failed a patient. Very many of the individual cases alleged have, on investigation, turned out either to be completely false or heavily distorted.' He then disappeared into the ether.

I stood against him in that election for the Struck Off and Die Junior Doctors' Alliance (SODJA), but I only met him at the count when he vaguely suggested we could meet up for a chat about my concerns (possibly knowing that he wouldn't be health secretary any more). The Bristol heart scandal was going on in his constituency, under his nose, but he was relieved to get out of the Department of Health relatively unscathed.

PRIVATE EYE

17 January 1992

It's an unhappy new year all round for those working in health secretary William Waldegrave's beleaguered NHS. . . .

In Bloomsbury, junior doctor Chris Johnstone has won the right to sue his health authority for subjecting him to a particularly onerous obstetrics job, and little progress has been made on cutting doctors' hours. Johnstone took his decision after falling asleep at the wheel. He used a portable brain-wave monitor to measure his cerebral activity during a 48-hour shift, and found that he was registering sleep waves while sewing up women after labour. Despite his high court victory, the job remained the same and the doctor who followed him spent time in intensive care after a paracetamol overdose.

The Government is trying to reduce junior doctors' hours in the most intensive jobs to just 83 per week without employing any more doctors. Forcing the same number of doctors to do the same amount of work in less time will be even more dangerous than the present system. The deal itself can only be saved if consultants agree to make up the shortfall in manpower. Meanwhile, a year after the deal was announced, surgical house officers in Newcastle are working 150 hours a week to cover for colleagues on holiday.

14 February 1992

In health secretary William Waldegrave's home city, managers at the United Bristol Healthcare Trust have come up with a novel way to cut waiting lists. Since all operations, however trivial, are counted together, list reductions have been achieved by concentrating on tiny plastic procedures. Lorry loads of 'bat ears', some of whom had been waiting for more than 10 years, were pinned back en masse at the expense of more substantial operations that took longer – a triumph of numbers over need.

With Mr Major's two-years-or-less waiting list promise looming, NHS managers are desperate to farm operations out to local private hospitals. Some private patients currently reach theatre without being examined and, with just one doctor resident in most private hospitals, the level of post-operative supervision is, er, not all it might be. And if shit happens, there isn't a cardiac arrest team close at hand. As many of the NHS patients are likely to be elderly, and a lot sicker than your average private patient, one can only hope that no-one suffers in this efficiency drive.

The current record for NHS understaffing is held by Manor Park Hospital, also in Bristol, where a single on-call junior doctor has to look after 360 geriatric in-patients, some of whom are very ill, sprawled over eighteen wards. Plymouth comes a close second, where one doctor is expected to minister to sick geriatric patients in three busy hospitals at once. The job includes the traditional 81-hour continuous shift, known locally as 'suicide weekend'.

Many NHS staff contracts have now been doctored to include an intimidating 'loyalty clause' effectively forbidding freedom of speech. Staff who do speak out are being shown the door. A leaked managerial document from Trent aimed to end the 'paranoia and posturing of rival professional groups' by sacking 'renegades and subversives.' Ouch.

In Cheltenham, the on-call room for the anaesthetist covering the intensive care unit has been helpfully moved to the far end of the hospital, well outside the two-minute emergency-sprinting distance. And down in the Special Care Baby Unit, senior house officers with no paediatric experience have no emergency back-up either, apart from a consultant-at-home. One junior was told he'd need to 'fly by the seat of his pants' if he got the job.

28 February 1992

The Royal Gwent in Newport, like many other district general hospitals, employs inexperienced junior doctors to cover the Special Care Baby Unit and labour wards with only a consultant-at-home for back-up. The unit turns over 4,500 babies a year, all of whom require oxygen to the brain well before the 30 minutes it takes a paediatrician to arrive in an emergency. One doctor was left alone to ventilate a 28-week-old baby on a new machine with an instruction manual in German. Meanwhile, in Chepstow, junior plastic surgeons are clocking up 100 hours a week, a mere ten years after attempts to abolish such rotas.

13 March 1992

The King's Fund's observation that London's health system is 'near collapse' is a tad at odds with William Waldegrave's rosy prediction. Many inner-London hospitals charge at least 30% extra for routine treatments to subsidise their large quota of emergency and super-specialist work. Not surprisingly, they aren't faring too well in the Tories' internal market and are desperate to save money.

Managers at the Royal London Hospital Trust have cut community psychiatric nursing and other essential services by £250,000 to bail out emergency work. At King's Hospital, some patients have been stuck in the corridor for 36 hours and a few have died-in-waiting. Understaffing of intensive care beds has long caused avoidable deaths as very sick patients are nursed on general wards without adequate observation.

Delayed admissions and inadequate in-patient care of cancer patients at London's St Bartholomew's Hospital has led to the resignation of Mr Jerry Gilmore, a senior cancer surgeon. And the low media profile of psychiatric patients has allowed Victorian asylums to be run down en masse. Hackney Hospital recently won an award for 'worst psychiatric hospital in Britain' and consultant Dr Niall Moore has volunteered to bulldoze it down. Unfortunately, lack of community care means the alternative for many psychiatric patients is to be knocked down on a zebra crossing.

Community care continues to suffer from its 'insensitivity to the market' (although it won't be long before managers are pricing empathy). At Bexley Hospital in Kent, the intended closure of Elmdene Alcoholic Unit would deprive the area of a vital centre for detoxification, education and support. There simply isn't any profit in it.

27 March 1992

When a BBC Radio Bristol reporter asked William Waldegrave how he felt about taking over as health secretary, his reply was telling: 'I'd rather be back in the Foreign Office.' Today, a glance at the hospitals in his Bristol West constituency will do little to change his mind.

Recent reports of Bristol Children's Hospital demanding a cash pledge from Worcester Royal Infirmary before allowing a critically injured child through its doors may have caused ructions in the national press, but for those working in Bristol, it hardly raised an eyebrow. The Bristol Royal Infirmary (BRI) has a long standing 'bed crisis' in intensive care because managers have persistently refused to provide the specialist staff needed to service more than five beds.

In the last four months, 94 patients have been refused an intensive care bed and 40% have subsequently died. Patients who have the misfortune to miss out are nursed on general wards, often by agency nurses with no specialist training. But despite the lack of beds, the rush to beat the April waiting-list deadline has meant that vascular surgeons are continuing to do major cases, such as aneurysm repairs, without post-operative intensive care.

On the weekend of February 22 and 23, the situation became farcical. The intensive care unit was again full. Two patients, surrounded by their distraught relatives, were artificially ventilated in the recovery room of an emergency operating theatre, blocking its use. Several other would-be intensive care patients were nursed on general wards and at least two requiring ventilation didn't get it. One patient who was bleeding from an ulcer would 'in an ideal world have had surgery', according to her doctor. She was denied it because she would have required intensive care post-op. Every surgeon has now received a memo asking them not to operate on any patient who may need intensive care afterwards.

THE OBSERVER
Junior, Behave Yourself

28 June 1992
Should you feel sorry for junior doctors? You don't see many of us with rickets. Most come from cosy professional backgrounds and go on to earn healthy sums of money in secure jobs with satisfaction and respect. And a few are so insufferably arrogant, it's hard for the rest to engender mass sympathy.

True, I could fill this column with horror stories of patients dying at the hands of tired, abused and unsupervised doctors, or of promising careers ending prematurely in alcoholism or suicide, but how much of that is self-inflicted? It's easy to blame 'the system' for a doctor's lot, but the system is largely composed of other doctors and we never were very good at accepting the buck. 'Bury the notes and burn the X-rays' is the stock solution to another tired cock-up.

After five years fighting a futile hours-reduction battle that started when I was in nappies, one question still perplexes me. How can a profession that purports to care for patients have so little regard for its own? The vast majority of consultants are not knowingly abusive towards their junior staff. True, there is a countrywide smattering of childishly malevolent surgeons who could do with an empathy infusion, but many more well-meaning specialists still suffer from a huge reality gap.

Most of us communicate badly with patients because we've never been poor, sick, black or even female. But even when we've experienced the iniquities of medical training first hand, it's all too easy to progress into consultant-hood with the misguided air of 'it didn't do me any harm.' Besides, if you've sacrificed your marriage and your liver to make it to the top, you don't want the bastards beneath you to find an easier route.

And after a few whiskies in the clubby locker-room atmosphere of an all-male common room, you tend to view your formative years through blood-tinted spectacles: 'We used to work for weeks on end … never saw daylight … and I enjoyed every minute of it.' Blah, blah, blah. Long hours weren't quite so onerous when the only therapeutic options were Horlicks or extra potatoes.

Technology, turnover and patient expectation have risen so sharply that few consultants have any idea what life's like on the bottom rung today. And with the administration, intimidation and uncertainty of the reforms, none of them has the stamina to find out.

Perhaps junior doctors deserve the mess they're in. Too many of us would rather sacrifice our own and our patients' well-being than stand up for ourselves. The combination of apathy, fear and fatigue has never allowed us to present a united front. 'Give us what we want or a handful of us will get in a strop' is unlikely to cut much ice with the Tories.

It would be nice to have a well-organised union behind us but we're stuck with the BMA. The traditional public school bias of medicine has bred a self-perpetuating profession of sheltered, spoon-fed sycophants with as much independent thought as a decerebrate baboon.

Though medical schools now accept students from a broader base, the mould remains to be broken: you don't see many black or female faces in a Royal College of Surgeons' group photo. Assured of success, the 'white, male and hearty' brigade have no need to rock the boat. Anyone else dare not. 'You're only as good as your last reference' is the familiar cry of the downtrodden doctor. Moving from job to job every six months, our futures depend on the vagaries of successive consultants. Tough luck if you end up with Sir Lancelot Spratt.

The only possible way out of this mess is for the profession to accept its share of the blame. The problem isn't simply one of hours. There's a long-standing cycle of self-inflicted abuse that has become so ingrained into junior doctor culture that even patients cease to be shocked by it.

The cycle will be impossible to break without a simultaneous overhaul of our training. The restrictive and secretive practices of the Royal Colleges must be replaced with openly restructured and team-based training, so that a whimsical prejudice doesn't mean the end of a promising career. Consultant selection must have more to do with clinical competence and less to do with trouser legs.

Training should be centred on one area, so doctors can establish a home base and a low-alcohol social life, and learn to fight their ground with consultants and managers alike. And working conditions should be well publicised so juniors can shop around for humane jobs while unpleasant ones remain unfilled.

None of this is likely to happen overnight. The Government, too, has become so blinkered that many long-term improvements are being sacrificed on the ill-advised altar of waiting lists *über alles*. But only tradition bars doctors from being supportive of each other. And if we swallowed our egos, we'd get a lot more sympathy.

Dr Phil's Notes

I've never totally recovered from my angry junior doctor phase, but it peaked after about five years. During that time, I was photographed dropping a baby for the *Sunday Times Magazine*, I threatened to take junior doctors out on strike in Jersey, I picketed the Tory conference in Blackpool and I stood for parliament against the health secretary William Waldegrave.

I took Waldegrave to the wire in Bristol West, creaming off 87 votes to his 22,169. In retrospect, hiring an ice-cream van as a campaign bus and driving around the streets of Clifton shouting 'What do we want? Willie Out! When do we want it? Now!' was never going to get me elected. The futility of using comedy to change anything was driven home by Harvey Thomas, Margaret Thatcher's campaign manager, who told me: 'You're a medical kook. If you want to be taken seriously, you have to be serious.' Doesn't seem to be working for Gordon Brown, though. You need optimism and a smile that doesn't frighten children too.

Comedy exists purely to make people laugh. You can't save the NHS with it, because you can never be sure why people are laughing. When I stood on stage at Edinburgh and said 'my local heart surgery unit is known as the Killing Fields and the Departure Lounge,' people roared with laughter. Doctors seemed to think it was particularly funny, and even if a few of them thought 'there's something not quite right going on there,' they weren't going to do anything about it. Their emotional response was to laugh, and having done that, they could move on to the next scary story.

Displacing your emotions into satire and black humour happens a lot in medicine. Every hospital has a surgeon known affectionately as 'Butcher' or 'Hacker' or even 'The Terminator'. Bristol boasted a heart surgeon called 'Killer' long before the heart scandal. But very few people blow the whistle or act to protect patients, although they might try to ensure their friends and family are diverted elsewhere. Even though Tony and I were outraged by our dangerous working conditions, I suspect *Struck Off and Die* reinforced as many attitudes as we changed. You can judge for yourself in a chapter tucked away near the end of *Medicine Balls*.

My medical hero is an American surgeon called Ernest Codman, who tried to change the world with passion and sincerity: 'I am called eccentric for saying in public that hospitals, if they wish to be sure of improvement, must find out what their results are, must analyse their results to find their strong and weak points, must compare their results with those of other hospitals, must care for what cases they can care for well, and avoid attempting to care for cases which they are not qualified to care for well. They must welcome publicity not only for their successes, but for their errors. Such opinions will not be eccentric a few years hence.' And that was in 1910.

Codman was, and still is, spot on. To have any idea if anything works in medicine, you have to measure outcomes and that means doing post-mortems on the dead to find out why they died, and talking to the living to find out if you've made any difference to their lives. The best part of *Struck Off and Die* was in the bar afterwards where other doctors would tell shocking stories we could nick, but patients too would share their experiences. Many loved the NHS, but some had a dreadful time. Slowly the penny dropped, and I shifted from defending doctors to protecting patients.

The pious *Observer* piece was deservedly rude about the medical establishment. I couldn't understand how a profession that was so intelligent and influential couldn't get its act together over junior doctors' hours. They have eventually come down (some say by too much), and the junior doctors who campaigned the hardest are now beleaguered consultants working harder than ever to cover their junior staff, who knock off as soon as their shift is over and complain they aren't getting enough training. But I hope we don't return to the dark days of 1992, when abused and exhausted juniors fell asleep in the wards.

VIRGINIA BOTTOMLEY
1992–1995

Gorgeous, pouting Virginia Hilda Brunette Maxwell Bottomley was known to her colleagues as Nanny, because of her fondness for health promotion. She saw her role as a custodian rather than a politician, to bed-in the Tory reforms: 'In politics you sometimes want a window-breaker and sometimes a glazier. Ken Clarke was definitely a window-breaker and I'm much more a glazier.'

She made the old farts in the British Medical Association swoon, and they gave her a standing ovation for instigating a deal to reduce junior doctors' hours (though not quickly enough for me). She also increased medical school numbers just before she left office. She didn't seem that keen on markets either, and in her valedictory speech, she extolled the virtues of planning and collaboration.

I've met her twice, once at the Hospital Doctor of the Year Awards in 1992, when she fretted that the winner might come from a London hospital that was earmarked for closure in the Tomlinson review. And once at a BUPA 60th Anniversary Celebration, when she didn't laugh at any of my jokes but I flogged her a couple of copies of *Medicine Balls* (replete with the unfortunate anagram of her name – I'm an evil Tory bigot).

Bottomley struck me as terribly earnest and well-meaning, but a bit too close to doctors, perhaps because she has them in her family. Like Waldegrave before her, she didn't seem to notice the Bristol heart scandal, even though parents wrote to her for advice in 1992. The Government could pour public money into a failing, dangerous service without taking any responsibility for the outcome.

The Bristol Heart Disaster
1992

Dr Phil's Notes

The Bristol heart disaster was one of the first stories I broke in *Private Eye* and it became the subject of the largest public inquiry in UK history, just seven years later. It finally forced the NHS to at least think about quality and safety, although this momentum was lost when they disappeared up the arse of Labour's competitive and secretive NHS market. At the time of writing, I didn't distinguish Bristol from any other example of dangerous care within the NHS. Thousands of people died (and still die) unnecessarily each year, and Bristol was only different in that it was babies rather than, say, old people.

Bristol hospitals were unfairly over-represented when I started writing for *Private Eye*, because I was living there and had lots of good sources. Only one has ever been brave enough to go public, the anaesthetist Stephen Bolsin, who paid for his concerns with his career and is now practising, very successfully, in Australia. Bolsin told the Bristol inquiry that he gave me information about the heart surgery unit as a concerned professional, and had no idea I wrote for *Private Eye*. So what follows is all my fault.

What vexed me in 1992 was not just that those in authority knew what was happening in Bristol and didn't act, but that the hospital management had the gall to pursue an award from the Department of Health while protecting a dangerous child heart surgery unit.

PRIVATE EYE

8 May 1992

Before the Department of Health bestows its mark of excellence on the United Bristol Healthcare Trust, it may wish to ponder the perilous state of its paediatric cardiac surgery. In 1988, the mortality was so high that the unit was dubbed 'The Killing Fields'. Despite a long crisis of morale among intensive care staff, the surgeons persistently refuse to publish their mortality rates in a manner comparable to other units. And although Dr Roylance (the chief executive) and the Department of Health are well aware of the problems, they won't recognise them officially.

Recently, the unit failed to provide a paediatric cardiac surgery nurse for post-operative care because it was assumed the baby would not survive the operation. And although Liverpool surgeons have successfully operated on 160 babies with Fallot's tetralogy, a congenital heart abnormality, the Bristol mortality rate is between 20% and 30%. Hardly the stuff of commendations.

3 July 1992

Health secretary Mrs Bottomley claims that whistle-blowing 'through the correct channels' will get results. Staff at the United Bristol Healthcare Trust (UBHT) have been whistling about the dismal mortality statistics in the paediatric cardiac surgery unit since 1988. And while UBHT's chief executive John Roylance, the Royal College of Surgeons and the NHS Management Executive are well aware of the problem, they seem more concerned with silencing the blowers.

In America, the mortality rate for arterial switch, an operation to connect congenitally transposed arteries from the heart is now 0%. Nearer to home in Birmingham it is 3%. In Bristol, despite the fact that the operation has been performed since 1988, it is 30%. Sadly, consultant cardiologists at the Bristol Children's Hospital continue to refer patients to their surgeons to support the local unit. As a recently retired and very eminent cardiac surgeon in Southampton says: 'Everyone knows about Bristol.'

9 October 1992

The sorry state of paediatric cardiac surgery at the United Bristol Healthcare Trust has been confirmed by an internal audit of the last two years' operations. The results of procedures to correct two congenital abnormalities (Tetralogy of Fallot and transposition of the arteries) were especially poor. James Wisheart, chairman of the hospital management committee and medical adviser to the Trust board, is required to maintain standards of medical practice at UBHT. Curiously he has not felt it necessary to inform the Trust board or the Trust's purchasers of these findings. Could it be because he is also associate director of cardiac surgery?

20 November 1992

At the Bristol Royal Infirmary, part of the United Bristol Healthcare Trust (UBHT), ward closures and patient transfers have made the surviving wards look full, thus giving the impression that business is booming. Such imaginative management has resulted in UBHT being awarded a charter mark, despite its precarious paediatric cardiac surgery unit. All-day celebrations were generously sponsored by the trustees and a commemorative lapel badge is being commissioned for staff to wear with pride. Curiously, UBHT just happens to be in the middle of former health secretary William Waldegrave's constituency.

Letter Printed in *Private Eye*

18 December 1992

Sir,

I see that you are having another swipe at Bristol Royal Infirmary's 'precarious' paediatric cardiac surgery unit. Exactly what your objections to this unit are escape me, but I feel moved to write in its defence. Our son, born with Down's syndrome and congenital heart disease, was operated on at BRI last November to repair his hole in the heart. Every member of the staff showed an unswerving dedication to all aspects of Joseph's operation, including helping us, his family, through the most traumatic experience we have ever known.

I have heard it suggested that some hospitals are not prepared to carry out such an operation if the child concerned has Down's syndrome, as the risk of failure is too high. (This may be only unfounded rumour, so is likely to appear as fact in your next issue, no doubt.) Since the majority of children with Down's syndrome have such a heart defect with associated operative risk, those hospitals that are prepared to carry out the operation may well appear way down the list in a league table of success v. failure. However, what is the true story behind the bald statistics? Leave the BRI, or at least the cardiac unit, alone. Without it and all its staff, our son would be ill and dying. He is fit and healthy only because of them.

Yours faithfully,
Jeremy Doyle
Kingswear, Dartmouth

Dr Phil's Notes

Although the Bristol unit enjoyed some success, the public inquiry concluded that a third of the children who underwent open-heart surgery between 1984 and 1995 received 'less than adequate care' and in one four-year period alone (1991 to 1995) 'between 30 and 35 more children under one year died after open-heart surgery in the Bristol Unit than might be expected had the Unit been typical of other Paediatric Cardiac Surgery units in England at the time.'

Bristol was an entirely avoidable tragedy. Had the surgeons taken note of Ernest Codman, concentrated on the simpler operations they could do well and referred the difficult operations to other units with the appropriate expertise, there would have been no scandal. Complex paediatric heart surgery needs specialist paediatric heart surgeons, and Bristol didn't have one. They had two adult surgeons in their mid-fifties trying to do the really hard stuff with staff shortages and shocking facilities. They should have recognised their own limitations during surgery, and instigated an inquiry after one unexpected death, not thirty-five. And when they refused to stop, the Department of Health and Royal College of Surgeons should have stepped in to stop them.

Private Eye didn't stop the surgeons either, but it certainly had an effect. In 1992, no UK surgeons were releasing their figures to the public and I guess that having them released for you in a satirical magazine, especially when they were this bad, might just piss you off rather than make you stop and think. Once you're in siege-mentality mode, it can be hard to break out of it and my exposure may just have contributed to that.

The public inquiry didn't report until 2001, which tells you how accountable the NHS was at that time, but they performed an impressive audit trail of the *Eye* articles which at least proved that everyone in authority knew about Bristol, and they might even have done something about it had the president of the Royal College of Surgeons not gone on holiday and missed a vital meeting at the Department of Health. The figures for Bristol stuck out like a sore thumb as far back as 1989, but while they remained unpublished, they could be hidden and parents were left in the dark. One *Eye*-reading couple did at least write to health secretary Virginia Bottomley to ask for her advice.

25 May 1992

> Dear Mrs Bottomley,
> We were disturbed to read in a recent edition of *Private Eye*, a report about the paediatric cardiology unit at Bristol. The column implies that a child undergoing surgery in Bristol stood less chance of surviving than in other parts of the country. Our child is due to have an operation in Bristol in the very near future, to try to alleviate a congenital heart defect. We have been warned that there is a one-in-four chance of failure and we are now concerned to know if the risk may be reduced if the operation were to take place elsewhere.

Just one month later, Ms J Binding, from Corporate Affairs at the NHS Management Executive at the Department of Health bounced the letter back to John Roylance, the chief executive at Bristol:

22 June 1992

> Dear Dr Roylance,
> The attached correspondence has just (sic) been received. It raises matters which can best be dealt

with by your Trust. I would be grateful if you could look into the matter and reply directly to [the parents]. I do not need to have a copy of your reply at this stage but I may need to ask for one later.

Clearly Mrs Bottomley and the NHS Management Executive weren't keen to get involved. The next reaction to the *Eye* came from Sir Keith Ross, an eminent retired cardiac surgeon from Southampton who had set up a Working Party to report to the Department of Health on units carrying out child heart surgery. He should have known what the Bristol figures were, so I was puzzled by the letter he wrote to senior Bristol heart surgeon, James Wisheart:

7 July 1992

Dear James,
I am writing to you in some distress because I have just been told of a comment about Bristol paediatric cardiac surgery, supposedly by someone who could only have been me by inference, in *Private Eye*. Please accept my complete and unqualified denial of any such comment – not only have I not discussed your unit with anyone outside the Working Party, I can honestly say I have no knowledge of your results. I can only assume that some malicious person who knows I sit on the Working Party has, for some reason best known to himself, seen fit to ascribe this comment to me. As always in this situation, there is nothing I can do except acquire an even deeper hatred of the behaviour of the press.
With kind regards,
Keith

Ross later admitted that he knew Bristol's overall figures were poor compared to other units, but didn't have a breakdown of individual operations. I was hoping the *Eye* might spur him into investigating, but he and Wisheart were old friends who had worked together. As Ross told the inquiry: 'James made a good impression as a conscientious and meticulous young surgeon ... we altogether enjoyed a satisfactory personal relationship and when my time finished on the Council of the British Heart Foundation, I had no hesitation in recommending him as my successor.' Ross could have been, but clearly wasn't, the man to support an investigation at Bristol.

However, the *Eye* nearly managed to get a result thanks to a letter from Dr John Zorab, a consultant anaesthetist and medical director at Frenchay Hospital in Bristol. He wrote to Sir Terence English, another eminent cardiac surgeon, immediate past-president of the Royal College of Surgeons and a member of the Department of Health's Advisory Group, which oversaw the provision and funding of paediatric cardiac surgery services.

15 July 1992

> Dear Terence,
> Sometime last autumn, I made one or two efforts to get to see you in order to discuss the delicate and serious problem of mortality and morbidity following paediatric cardiac surgery in Bristol. Great anxieties were being expressed by some of my colleagues at the Royal Infirmary. In the event, I never made contact and the matter passed from the forefront of my mind.
>
> Matters have come to a head once again and the enclosed piece from *Private Eye*, whilst possibly having some inaccuracies, quotes some statistics

that have been confirmed elsewhere. One of the newer consultant cardiac anaesthetists feels that the mortality rate is too distressing to be tolerated and is job-hunting elsewhere.

Whether the *Eye* is correct in saying that the matter has already been drawn to the attention of the College and the NHS Management Executive, I do not know. There is, however, a widespread feeling that the situation is well-recognised but being ignored – possibly because no-one knows how to tackle it.

Yours sincerely
John

Again, this letter shouldn't have been too much of a surprise. Back in 1989, Ross's Working Party reported to the Advisory Group that Bristol had a higher mortality rate than the other units. The medical secretary of the Advisory Group, Dr Norman Halliday, told the inquiry that when Bristol was given the Department of Health's seal of approval to operate on babies and children in 1984, it 'did not actually shine like a star' and 'performance was not on a par with other units.'

The hope was that performance would somehow improve. It didn't. In October 1986, Professor Andrew Henderson of the University of Wales distributed a letter at a meeting of South Glamorgan Health Authority stating: 'it is no secret that their [Bristol's] paediatric cardiac surgery service is regarded as being at the bottom of the UK league for quality.' Dr Halliday was informed but felt he could not take the case further as no supporting evidence was attached.

In 1989, Halliday received the Working Party report outlining poor outcomes in Bristol and, in 1990, he visited the unit and noted 'sub-optimal' results, attributed to the low volume of work. In February 1992, Dr Halliday was handed

Bristol's very poor 1991 figures but he 'didn't have the machinery to analyse the data'.

Bristol was a well-known and long-standing problem that should have been sorted out long before *Private Eye* put it in the public domain in 1992. Dr Zorab's letter convinced Sir Terence English to 'revisit the 1991 figures on mortality'. He now realised that the Bristol unit stood out as far worse than anywhere else, even though the Working Party had recommended that it should carry on. In his reply to Zorab, English wrote:

27 July 1992

> Dear John
> . . . I will make a full response when I return from holiday in mid-August. Suffice it to say at this stage Bristol is not included in the paediatric cardiac surgical units recommended by the Royal College of Surgeons for continued designation for supra-regional funding. The Working Party report will be considered by the Advisory Group on 28th July.
> Yours sincerely
> Terence

So although Ross's Working Party had recommended that Bristol be allowed to continue despite the bad results, the Advisory Group was going to overrule and recommend funding be withdrawn, which would stop the surgeons operating. Alas, English was off on holiday and would miss the vital meeting, but he agreed this plan of action with Professor David Hamilton, a colleague from the Royal College of Surgeons who would be attending. And he wrote a letter to Professor Norman Browse, who had just replaced him as president of the Royal College of Surgeons:

24 July 1992

> Dear Norman,
> ... In the [Working Party] report, which is to be considered on 28th July, Bristol was included as one of the centres for designation. However, it is clear from a review of the report that their mortality statistics, both for the infant age group and the older age group, are worse than any other centre. David Hamilton agrees that sufficient attention was not paid to this by his Working Party. We agreed, therefore, that to allow Bristol to go forward with support from the College might jeopardise designation of the whole service and, with David's agreement, I have spoken to Norman Halliday who will inform the Advisory Group on Tuesday, 28th that the College does not support the inclusion of Bristol; I am sure this is the right action.
> Yours sincerely
> Terence

Private Eye, thanks to John Zorab, had got the Royal College of Surgeons to see sense. Or it might have done had Sir Terence not been in Pakistan. When he returned, there was a letter waiting for him from Professor David Hamilton:

3 August 1992

> Dear Terence,
> I hope that you had a highly successful trip to and safe journey back from Pakistan, and are refreshed after a demanding but successful term as President. Following our telephone conversations of

Thursday evening, July 23rd, and Friday afternoon, 24th, I was not entirely happy about our agreement to take action over the Working Party's report. On reflection, I realised a possible specific source of breach of confidentiality which could arise and a further feeling that the de-designation of one of the units would probably leak out in the course of time.

Also, the members of the Working Party were unanimous in their findings and gave considerable thought to their recommendations. Like you, I was unable to contact Keith Ross, but did so early on Monday morning, the 27th, after he had returned home from holiday. He was equally concerned that we had changed the report and suggested on reflection that we should both speak with Norman Halliday to reverse the decision and the instruction that you had given him.

. . . The Working Party could be requested by the Advisory Group to reconsider the mortality figures of specific units (or unit) and possibly to amend its findings. This appealed to me as a far safer course of action.

Yours sincerely

David

Safer for whom? The Advisory Group refused to take action against Bristol to protect babies from unnecessary death because the data from all units had been collected in confidence and if Bristol was 'struck off', it would be obvious that it was the one with the really bad results that stuck out like a sore thumb (and which everyone knew was Bristol anyway). Such was the mindset in 1992. And, as Keith Ross pointed out, there was an unfortunate holiday clash:

When David Hamilton phoned me, I had just returned from Scotland and had no idea of the events leading up to the telephone call ... I must have agreed with his concern regarding the Working Party's conclusions being altered but there was no way I could have talked to Terence English as he was either in, or on his way to, Pakistan. ... In fact, the convergence of so many factors at the end of July 1992, which included Dr Zorab's letter, a new President of the Royal College of Surgeons and the absence of Sir Terence English (and for that matter myself) from the Advisory Group meeting was a historical disaster.

Ross's Working Party never revisited Bristol's mortality figures. English told the inquiry that he specifically raised them with Dr Halliday, but Halliday disputed this. The matter was never even raised at any future Advisory Group meeting, even though they were both members. The high death rates were not investigated and Bristol continued unchecked until the death of Joshua Loveday three years later.

By 1995, the surgeons had supposedly agreed to stop the more complex operations until a specialist paediatric cardiac surgeon was appointed. But they pressed ahead with Joshua's surgery despite opposition from anaesthetic staff, other surgeons and the Department of Health. Joshua died, the shit hit the fan and the rest of the media finally cottoned on. Even the General Medical Council (GMC) woke up and instigated one of the biggest arse-covering operations in the history of medicine.

Why did no-one step in earlier? As Bristol inquiry chairman Ian Kennedy observed with some anger: 'One of the features of our taking evidence is that no matter whom we have spoken to – whether it be a health authority, a trust, a royal college and now a department [of health] – they have always found someone else responsible.' His comments were in response to the evidence of Sir Graham Hart, a permanent secretary at the Department of Health until 1997. In Sir Graham's view: 'Ministers who are politicians should not be involved in the clinical treatment of patients,' and there was a 'deeply rooted reserve' against the department becoming involved in monitoring clinical performance.

Doctors can't have it all their own way. If they want to regulate themselves and not have politicians interfering in clinical matters, they have to be open about their results. Publication of outcomes is essential to maintain trust, as is sound statistical analysis to identify a 'significant outlier' that needs swift investigation. And politicians, civil servants and managers shouldn't just plough money into a failing service in the vain hope it will get better.

Kennedy later referred to the process of designating which centres should perform child heart surgery as having 'all the qualities of a Greek tragedy. . . . Bristol was frankly not up to the task. . . . There is real room for doubt as to whether open heart surgery on the under-1s should have been designated in Bristol.' The inquiry tried very hard not to blame anyone but concluded that 'in certain respects, when concerns were raised, in the roles they then occupied, Dr Halliday and Sir Terence English should have behaved differently.'

When I gave evidence to the inquiry, I was vaguely threatened with a custodial sentence for not revealing all my sources. (I realised then that I probably should have brought a lawyer along.) I then received a warning letter saying that the inquiry might criticise me for raising concerns in *Private Eye* rather than 'the usual channels' but they backed off, presumably when they realised how ineffectual the Royal College of Surgeons and the Department of Health were.

The General Medical Council (motto: 'Protecting patients, guiding doctors') wasn't much use either. Having failed to protect any babies, they jumped in before the public inquiry to save face and pin the disaster on three doctors: the two surgeons, James Wisheart and Janardan Dhasmana, and the hospital chief executive John Roylance, who was also a doctor.

Roger Henderson, QC for the GMC, left little room for doubt: 'Mr Wisheart should have realised by 1993 that the mortality of up to 54% associated with the operations he carried out to correct atrioventricular septal defects – compared with the national average of 13.9% – was comparatively disastrous.' But the GMC didn't define statistically what it meant by 'comparatively disastrous'. Twice as bad as the national average? Three times? Four times? Unless you set this safety standard, there is no automatic trigger to tell surgeons to stop operating and start investigating.

Wisheart had voluntarily stopped operating before the GMC inquiry. An external assessment of his adult surgery between January 1993 and September 1995 found that his 30-day death rate for lower-risk arterial bypass operations was 12.2% versus an average of other consultants of 2.6%. When it came to all coronary artery bypass operations, Wisheart's death rates were 13.4%, compared to the average of 4.1%. He was described by the auditors as 'a higher risk surgeon' with a performance that 'appeared to be significantly poorer than the others.' He'd gone off the boil all round, hardly surprising given the stress he was under.

The GMC found that the two surgeons 'had continued to perform certain operations despite growing concerns about poor mortality figures. They did not adequately establish the causes of those results. One of them misled parents about likely outcomes. And the then chief executive failed to take action when colleagues voiced anxieties.' In 1998, the GMC struck off Wisheart (who had retired) and Roylance, and suspended Dhasmana (whose adult figures were good) from carrying out child heart surgery for three years.

The GMC is very good at punishing doctors long after the event, but its claim to protect patients has never quite stacked up. Until he retired, Dr Michael O'Donnell was the longest-serving member of the GMC and chairman of its professional standards committee. In a statement to the inquiry, he wrote: 'Over lunch at a GMC council or committee meeting, I'd raised the subject of what seemed to be happening in Bristol, almost certainly prompted by what I'd read in *Private Eye*. Though one or two of the people I discussed it with seemed concerned, the general reaction was one of intense apathy.'

Five years later, when the GMC was forced into action, O'Donnell 'got a number of phone calls from doctors in and around Bristol who hadn't realised I was no longer on the GMC, wanting me to know what a good chap Wisheart was and wondering if I could "do anything" to get the charges dropped. One of the callers assured me, rather alarmingly, that someone in the past had managed to "do something" about another case.'

O'Donnell also revealed details of two GMC health screeners 'who had to decide if a doctor's ability to practise might be impaired by any illness or alcohol dependency. The pair were known to have "drinking problems" and yet were allowed to remain in office. . . . I raised my concern about the first screener with the then president. The problem with the second was so widely known that the secretariat tried to ensure that alcohol was not available at midday during meetings of the Health Committee.'

The journalist in me is very good at exposing scandals in black and white in under 800 words, but it took a public inquiry lasting two and a half years, with evidence from 577 witnesses and 900,000 pages of documents to make sense of what happened in Bristol in the broader context of a ludicrously underfunded and overburdened health service. The report of the inquiry, chaired by Ian Kennedy, is one of the wisest documents ever written about the NHS, and had its 198 recommendations been followed, the NHS would be a safe place to be sick in and I wouldn't be writing this book now. You can still access the report at www.bristol-inquiry.org.uk

The report points out that 'the story of the paediatric cardiac surgical service at Bristol is not an account of bad people. Nor is it an account of people who did not care, nor of people who wilfully harmed patients.' This was why they were so hard to stop. They weren't depressed or alcoholic or psychotic, they were workaholics. They should have stopped, but their unit would have lost funding and prestige. So they carried on.

The surgeons' supporters, and there are many, point out that their commitment and dedication were beyond doubt, the majority of their operations went well and that the biggest factor in their downfall was the understaffing and inadequate facilities they had to contend with. While these were indeed appalling, the inquiry stressed: 'It is crucial to make clear the following. The inadequacy of resources for paediatric cardiac surgery at Bristol was typical of the NHS as a whole. From this, it follows that whatever went wrong in Bristol was not caused by lack of resources. Other centres laboured under the same or similar difficulties. For example, the shortage of qualified nurses and cardiologists was a national phenomenon, affecting all centres. We therefore emphasise the point again that, while under-funding blighted the NHS as a whole, it does not alone provide the explanation for what went wrong at Bristol.'

The inquiry noted that the Bristol team showed a lack of insight and teamwork, poor communication and flawed behaviour. Hardly a recipe for safety. To perform paediatric cardiac surgery successfully, you need a functional team at the top of its game. I doubt my *Private Eye* articles helped teamwork or morale, not least because they spread mistrust: 'Which of you bastards has been speaking to the press?'

When I gave evidence to the inquiry, I said that the Bristol surgeons were fall guys for a much wider problem in the NHS – a complete lack of accountability. All doctors were pretty much free to do what they wanted, guided only by their clinical judgement, and that's a pretty dodgy compass. I didn't quote Codman, but I called for all surgical teams to have their outcomes measured, adjusted for risk and published. If the NHS provided a truly good service, this would restore trust and confidence. If it didn't, we needed to act.

Heart surgeons were first to grab the nettle. Since publication, mortality rates are continuing to fall and there's no evidence that sicker patients are being denied surgery. But the rest of the NHS remains a big black hole that we're only slowly shining a torch into now. As Kennedy pointed out on July 18, 2001: 'Even today, it is still not possible to say, categorically, that events similar to those which happened in Bristol could not happen again in the UK; indeed are not happening at this moment.' And we still don't know, eight years later.

More Scandals on the Bottomley Watch

PRIVATE EYE

16 February 1994

The inadequate resuscitation facilities in Liverpool hospitals first highlighted by sacked nursing student Kenneth MacDonald in 1991 have been further exposed in the *British Medical Journal* (*BMJ*). MacDonald complained that whilst working at Walton and Fazakerley hospitals, two patients were left to die when the cardiac arrest ('crash') team should have been called. The *BMJ* study of 297 patients at Fazakerley Hospital found that nearly a third of these were deemed not for resuscitation (NFR) by the medical staff (usually in the absence of a consultant) and in only a third of these cases had the prognosis been discussed with relatives. Nurses and doctors were sometimes unable to agree on whether to resuscitate, with the result that for five patients, the nurse didn't call the crash team even though the doctor wanted them to. MacDonald believes that such cases could be tantamount to manslaughter and has asked the Mersey constabulary to investigate.

20 February 1994

Mrs Bottomley's dubious defence of community psychiatric care in the wake of the Clunis Report centred on a small increase in the number of community psychiatric nurses (CPNs). At present, there are 5,000 such nurses and six million people with mental health problems. For schizophrenia alone, only one person in five has access to a CPN and there are likely to be at least a hundred patients as disturbed as Christopher Clunis, who stabbed Jonathan Zito to death at Finsbury Park tube in 1992, walking around London at the moment. Ironically, it was the public outcry over lack of community supervision of such disturbed patients which initially led to the construction of long-stay psychiatric hospitals, many of which have now been closed (and sold off for housing). The report has asked for an urgent increase in the number of medium-secure beds in south-east London, where 45% of GPs have no access to mental health professionals whatsoever, and more general psychiatric beds in inner London.

How should doctors deal with violent patients? Stoke GP Dr Kauser Jafri has admitted to carrying an imitation .38 Smith and Wesson revolver in his doctor's bag for the last seventeen years for 'confidence and personal safety.' When faced with 'a drunk drug addict who was menacing and swore,' Dr Jafri found it particularly useful: 'I tried to appear calm but a chill ran down my spine. "Let me just examine you," I said very deliberately as I opened my bag. I took out my stethoscope slowly giving him the chance to see my revolver. The effect was stunning. His whole demeanour changed and I was able to send him away with just one day's supply of drugs.'

24 March 1994

Last year, anaesthetist Behrooz Irani was struck off after he switched off alarms on anaesthetic equipment at Humberside's Castle Hill Hospital and left a patient, who turned blue and had no heart beat for seven minutes, in a permanent vegetative state. Now the chairman of the anaesthetic division of East Yorkshire NHS Trust has been found guilty of serious professional misconduct by the GMC for failing to relieve Irani of his duties despite a number of warnings from senior operating department assistants.

Irani previously worked at Hull Royal Infirmary, where consultant surgeon Mr Alan Wilkinson had to administer artificial respiration to bring one of his patients round after the anaesthetic. Mr Wilkinson told the GMC hearing that 'the man was not safe' but added: 'In Hull we do not have consultant anaesthetists growing on trees. I didn't make a formal complaint because it was either him or nobody. We are constantly having to do that because we are so understaffed.' After leaving Yorkshire, Dr Irani worked as a locum in Chepstow, Gwent, until he was sacked after leaving a patient, whose oxygen level was dangerously low, to make a telephone call.

10 June 1994

Junior doctor Alan Massie died in January after working a continuous 86-hour shift in obstetrics and gynaecology at Warrington District General Hospital, just three years after the BMA and Mrs Bottomley decided that such stressful, unrelenting jobs should convert to a shift system, with no doctor working a longer stint than eight hours. The tribute to Dr Massie from the nursing staff at his funeral read: 'Always smiling, always tired, always hungry.'

18 August 1994

All is not well at Royal Oldham Hospital. Ten junior doctors have written to trust chairman Mary Firth claiming that 'gross understaffing' on the medical wards has led to 'dangerously inadequate levels of care.' Patients have to wait hours to be assessed by a doctor and the trust had to close to emergencies on several occasions in June and July. The elderly ward is staffed at half the recommended level, causing 'an impossible situation for the remaining on-call staff. The attention given to individual patients is desperately lacking on a day-to-day basis, and their admission stay is undoubtedly prolonged beyond what is necessary.' As Ms Firth observed: 'This is just a little blip.'

25 March 1995

'Institutions,' claimed Bertrand Russell, 'are to be judged by the good or harm they do to individuals.' The latest Office of Population Censuses and Surveys figures show that nurses top the league for female suicides, with 153 ending it all between 1990 and 1992. The second most at-risk group is female doctors and indeed seven of the top ten high-risk groups are professions related to medicine.

6 July 1995

Mrs Bottomley's last-gasp announcement as health secretary that the intake to medical schools is to be increased by 10% by the year 2000 may have come too late to solve the medical manpower crisis. It costs the taxpayer £192,000 to train a medical graduate, but up to a quarter of newly qualified doctors now give up or disappear abroad. Many parts of the NHS only function thanks to the efforts of overseas doctors, who occupy 26% of the training grades. In some specialties such as anaesthetics, psychiatry, paediatrics and general practice, there are often no applicants for jobs advertised in the

British Medical Journal. Increasing the student intake is unlikely to have any effect if the working conditions remain so poor. As one of this year's Birmingham graduates put it: 'When I first went on the wards in 1992, all the junior doctors told me to give up now and all the consultants said it would be alright in the end. Now everyone's telling me to get out.'

Just as alarming is the national shortage of consultants. There are 150 national consultant vacancies in anaesthetics alone, with trusts resorting to head-hunting, poaching, overseas recruitment and inflated salaries to fill posts. Dr Julia Moore, clinical director of anaesthetics at Merseyside's Wirral Trust, claims trusts are no longer advertising vacancies in the UK because they know there'll be no replies. As health minister Gerry Malone put it: 'I disagree with the words "manpower crisis."'

STEPHEN DORRELL
July 1995–May 1997

Stephen Dorrell is probably best known for wearing a chunky-knit, cuddle-me sweater to one of William Hague's informal love-ins, but his time as health secretary was marked by the fag end of the Major government and the emergence of two scandals, BSE and Bristol. No wonder he looked like a man tortured by irritable bowel syndrome.

In March 1996, Dorrell told the Commons that it was likely that the first ten cases of a rare brain disease called new variant CJD were due to exposure to beef products contaminated with BSE. Measures to prevent transmission of BSE to humans had been introduced back in 1988–89, so this shouldn't have been a news story. Bad luck then that every paper led with 'Mad Cow Killer' headlines and everyone stopped eating beef apart from John Gummer, the agriculture minister, who force-fed his daughter a burger for the camera. No-one would import British beef, farmers were rushed into the mass slaughter and burning of cherished herds and £3 billion went in compensation for what was essentially a non-scare. As Dorrell told Radio 4: 'It's not the cows that are mad, it's the public.' Clearly he was courting the dead cow vote.

Bristol emerged as a public scandal in 1995, and Dorrell ordered an inquiry. But it was left to Frank Dobson to decide whether to make it public, or to keep hiding the bad stuff.

PRIVATE EYE
New Wine in Old Bottles

4 August 1995

This October heralds the start of a huge country wide change in undergraduate medical education, with the introduction of the GMC's 'new' curriculum. Instead of cramming two hundred medical students into a sweaty lecture theatre or sending them off to cut up dead humans and live domestic mammals, they will now have their values explored in small focus groups before being dispatched into the community to learn about real life. Or so the theory goes.

The changes have met with a lot of resistance, principally from those who stand to lose financially. It costs the taxpayer £34,000 a year to train a medical student, so a medical school with a thousand students rakes in £34 million a year. Only a fraction of this has ever gone on teaching, with professors preferring to use the money to tart up their departments and conduct research. A typical surgical unit in a teaching hospital might receive £4 million a year in teaching money, and in return will allow a few students a week to tag onto the end of a ward round or hang on the end of a surgical instrument. Disciplines such as anatomy, physiology and biochemistry stand to lose most as the factual content of the course is slashed and replaced by subjects such as 'How We Learn' and 'Real People, Real Problems'.

The biggest problem facing medical education is not, however, the course content but the 'see one, do one, teach one' ethos of British medicine. Very few medical teachers are taught to teach, preferring to rely on their innate abilities. This, coupled with the patronage system that prevents juniors from complaining, has allowed many eminent consultants to humiliate their students over the years without fear of reprisal.

One consultant general surgeon at Birmingham's Selly Oak

Hospital prides himself on his amusing banter over the operating table. As a female student put it: 'First he asked me if I was from the home counties. When I said yes, he started calling me Tinkerbell and said I looked the sort of girl who'd had a horse between my legs. Then he asked me if I'd lost my virginity up against the wall of a horsebox while my mother was outside watching a gymkhana. The surgical registrar and the other theatre staff started laughing too. It was like being in a monkey house. At the end, he asked me if I minded him being sexist in theatre: "Women like to know what men want." Then he made a hole in the gall-bladder and said: "Look what you've made me do."'

Another consultant surgeon at the Queen Elizabeth Hospital was recently forced to apologise in writing to a female student after saying, 'You must have felt testicles before. Haven't you got a boyfriend?' Changing the curriculum without changing the attitudes of the staff could be disastrous. As Stanislaw Lec put it: 'If you give a cannibal a fork, is it progress?'

Pill Scare

20 October 1995
'I am acutely aware that this new information will worry women, and impose a substantial burden on doctors and pharmacists.' So said Professor M D Rawlins, chairman of the Government's Committee on the Safety of Medicines (CSM), in his letter informing every GP in the UK that seven of the most popular oral contraceptives should be abandoned for women with risk factors for venous thrombo-embolism such as obesity, varicose veins or a previous history of thrombosis of any cause. 'Other women,' concludes Rawlins, 'should continue to take them only if they are intolerant of other oral contraceptives and prepared to accept the increased risk of thrombo-embolism.'

Unfortunately, this information reached me twenty-four hours after it hit the press and not in time to reassure a surgery full of women, most of whom had no notion of the absolute and relative risk. The overall odds of a non-smoking under-35-year-old woman dying as a result of taking the pill are 1 in 77,000. For a pill-taking smoker under the age of 35, the odds are 1 in 10,000. The non-smoker is thirteen times more likely to die while driving a car, six times more likely to die as a result of pregnancy and two and a half times more likely to die in a household accident than from taking the pill. Two themes emerge: death on the pill is rare and if you want to reduce your risk, stopping smoking is far more important than which pill you take.

As for the risk of vein clots, these in themselves are inconvenient but only dangerous if the clot breaks off and bungs up the lungs. Venous thrombosis occurs in 1 in 10,000 non-pill-takers every year. Pill-takers were thought to have a 2 in 10,000 risk, but Professor Rawlins seems to be suggesting that those taking any of the magnificent seven may have a 3 in 10,000 risk. As 70% of the women in our practice are on these 'harmful' contraceptives, I wanted more evidence than a flimsy circular from the CSM before embarking on the wholesale disruption of their family planning.

This would not seem unreasonable, since this Government is constantly exhorting the value of evidence-based medicine, a founding principle of which is that grass-roots doctors should not accept the judgement of detached academics, but evaluate the evidence at first hand from the original scientific papers. This is even more important when an author of one of the papers, Professor Walter Spitzer, strongly disagrees with the CSM's interpretation. Earlier this year, the Government tried to blacklist these newer contraceptives on financial grounds, so I was naturally anxious that this might be part of the hidden agenda. Fortunately, Professor Rawlins' letter ended: 'If you require any further information, please call.'

When I phoned to ask for copies of the three unpublished papers on which this advice is based, I was told: 'You are not allowed to see the evidence.' When I pointed out that this was for my personal analysis of the validity and reliability of the studies in question, the phone went dead. Why should the trials be kept secret from doctors? At present, all I have is dozens of worried women and two Sainsbury's bags full of returned Marvelon and Femodene. Any offers?

Unkind Cuts

6 December 1995

'It is pointless to perform major surgery on patients who are physiologically compromised unless there are facilities for those patients to recover post-operatively.' So said the fourth annual *Independent National Enquiry into Perioperative Deaths in England, Wales and Northern Ireland.* Of the doctors surveyed, 81% had access to intensive care beds but only 21% had access to high-dependency units, which closely monitor patients who are still too sick to return to a general ward.

Lowlights of the 19,816 deaths that occurred within 30 days of operation include a 70-year-old man who underwent emergency surgery to repair a strangulated hernia, only to find the recovery room was closed for the night (he died 15 hours later) and a 54-year-old man who was admitted to a university hospital with a head injury. There were no neurosurgery beds available and the CT scanner was out of commission, delaying the diagnosis. When the need to operate was spotted, the two specialists were busy opening someone else's skull, resulting in a 5-hour delay. He died 16 days later.

A Junior Doctor Writes

18 January 1996

Dear Sir

I am a house officer at Wansbeck General Hospital, an institution that has featured several times in your column. Despite having been a doctor for only five months, I consider myself hardened, cynical and brutalised. I have seen my interests and hobbies decimated and have lost touch with friends because of my job. In February, I move to a trust in Sunderland, where my contract has been vetted and declared 'totally unacceptable' by the BMA's industrial relations officer. In August, I will join the hordes of junior doctors fleeing Britain to New Zealand, Australia and South Africa because I cannot envisage doing 3–4 more years as a senior house officer, working for these disgusting institutions.

At Wansbeck, a trust millions in debt, we admitted medical emergencies to surgical wards almost every day over Christmas and New Year. This is distressing for the nurses, who are not used to this type of patient, and bad for patients themselves who can easily be forgotten. On one weekday following New Year, 18 of 21 emergency medical admissions between 17.00 and 09.00 went to surgical wards, and a ward had to be re-opened to cope with demand. At the moment, the plan is to cut the number of medical beds despite year-round bed-occupancy rates well over 90%. The only thing that has made the job bearable is the 'in the trenches' camaraderie amongst junior doctors.

If you use any of the above, please don't mention my name. As you know, medicine is a patronage system and seems very sinister from where I am.

A Patient Writes

13 February 1996

Dear Sir,

Being disabled in my late forties, I wear a calliper on my leg and cannot walk far because I suffer from angina and asthma. Last Tuesday, I was admitted to the East Surrey Hospital at 9pm with an asthma attack. I was told that there were no beds available and that I would have to stay in the casualty department until one became free. After four hours on a hard trolley, I had an X-ray taken before being put to sleep in a very noisy plaster room. Next day, I thought I would be transferred to a ward. Not so. In fact, I was kept in the casualty department for three days and three nights, after which I was completely exhausted.

There was nowhere to wash, except in a small hand bowl, and just one toilet nearby. There wasn't enough bed linen and twice I had my pillow taken away from me when I left it. The noise was unbearable and the food arrived at 6pm and 8am, with nothing in-between. One night I was woken by a nurse trying to take my oxygen supply for another patient, and another nurse remonstrating with him saying that I needed it.

It's not the fault of the medical and nursing staff that these appalling conditions prevail. Indeed I feel sorry for them as all the time they were rushed off their feet. Their morale is at its absolute lowest. The nursing staff suggested that if I was not happy I should write and complain, as their grievances are constantly ignored and they can do little or nothing to get improvements. Who is to blame for all this? Is it just a lack of funds or what? It certainly needs sorting out.

Yours sincerely,
Mrs Gwen B Ross

A Relative Writes

6 June 1996

My father reached Princess Alexandra Hospital (Harlow) by emergency ambulance at 12.45pm on February 12, following a phone call from his GP stipulating that hospital admission was essential. On arrival, a notice board in reception informed us that we could expect a 3-hour wait due to staff sickness. My father was wheeled on an ambulance trolley into a draughty corridor where my mother and I waited with him for two hours. During that time, a nurse took his pulse, temperature and blood pressure, and gave him an oxygen mask. However, despite his obviously deteriorating condition and our repeated request for further examination, none was forthcoming. At 2.45pm he was allocated a cubicle, but was not seen by a doctor until 6.45pm.

The doctor who eventually examined him said that he was extremely dehydrated, which came as no great surprise as my mother and I had repeatedly expressed our concern to several members of staff that he was unable to tolerate any food or drink for over two days. However, we were told that no food or drink could be administered prior to being seen by a doctor. Before any action was taken to rehydrate him, he had to endure a series of X-rays when he was clearly in severe distress and lapsing into unconsciousness. By the time a drip bag was produced at 7.15pm, it took ten minutes to locate a drip stand. His oxygen tank was replaced, but only after I pointed out that it was empty. The soap dispenser in the cubicle was empty and no pillow could be found to support his head.

At 10pm, the doctor we had previously seen informed us that a line would have to be inserted into my father's neck, and politely asked us to wait outside. Several doctors came and emerged shortly afterwards to tell us he required urgent renal dialysis. My father was transferred to the Royal London Hospital at 11pm after a further delay due to a non-starting ambulance and a failure to locate some jump leads. On arrival at the Royal London, he was immediately allocated a bed and dialysis was commenced. This was unsuccessful and he was again transferred, to the intensive care unit at Bart's Hospital, where he died without regaining consciousness.

My father suffered from a serious illness, but had he received prompt medical treatment he would have at least been able to say his last goodbyes to us. Our devastation and heartbreak would have been terrible in any event without this additional burden to bear. I have since obtained a copy of the Patients' Charter for the people of North Essex which states that patients can expect to be treated with 'dignity and privacy' and that the 'care environment will be quiet, warm and comfortable'. This was not the case. He also has 'a right to emergency medical treatment at any time in the A&E department' but no timescales are mentioned, which merely compounds my cynicism.

A Consultant Writes

30 June 1996
Letter from Dr J E Carty, consultant rheumatologist, Lincoln and Louth NHS trust

For some time there has been a developing inequality between the services we provide to (non-fundholding) GPs through the Lincolnshire health contract and those to GP fundholders. Whilst there is no difference in the treatment and clinical decisions we make about patients, the access time for surgery is now a cause for great concern. There were many worries when GP fundholding was established that there would be a two-tier system: that certainly exists and in fact we have a several-tier system, with some fundholders seeking non-urgent surgery within three months and most within the 9–12 months range. For non-fundholders, we only guarantee the Patients' Charter Standards of 15 months for hips, knees and cataracts, and 18 months for everything else.

To give an example, one of my colleagues has undertaken the sterilisation and removal of a coil for a fundholder patient who has been waiting no more than 6 weeks, but is not able to give treatment to a Lincolnshire health patient with a fibroid uterus and debilitating heavy periods until mid-1997. This is unsettling and causing professional concern. We wish to treat patients on the basis of clinical need and not by virtue of the accident of where they live and the practice they are signed up with. This is supposed to be a National Health Service funded by universal taxation.

A Manager Writes

Letter from Tracey Baggott, contracts manager for GP Fundholders at Southampton University Hospitals NHS Trust

Due to financial pressures, some health authorities have had to take the difficult decision to impose service restrictions within their contracts and allow the waiting times for their residents to move out beyond previous targets. In order to manage this difficult situation, I am writing to request that all general practitioners could indicate on their referral letters to this Trust whether they are fundholders or not, for example by putting GPFH under their signature. This would enable the Trust to prioritise patients, if applicable. This will also help avoid consultants being placed in an awkward position whereby they are unsure whether the patient belongs to a fundholding practice or is the responsibility of the health authority, and will allow the consultant to give his patient a more accurate estimate of their expected waiting time.

Dr Phil's Notes

After twelve years in power, we're all keen to give Labour a good kicking, but looking back on my time under the Tories shows how they failed to make the NHS safer or sort out variable standards in care (and access to it). They introduced a management structure obsessed with money and efficiency without any responsibility for safety and quality. In such a system, danger thrived.

BLAME LABOUR
1997–

BLAME LABOUR
1997–

In opposition, Labour got NHS staff on their side by deriding the Tories' internal market as iniquitous and wasteful, and pledging to dismantle it. In office, they embraced it wholeheartedly, but not before ditching GP fundholding. The scheme was clearly unfair in that patients from these practices got quicker care than those from practices that were too small to qualify, or had ideological objections. But the danger of enforced equality is that it breeds mediocrity. The NHS needs room for innovation, even if some patients get it before others. Many fundholding GPs were both innovative and wise, grouping together to provide a whole range of services closer to patients' homes. They could also bypass hospitals if they had concerns about the quality and safety of care.

Twelve years of Labour and a vast sum of public money later, the English NHS is stuck with a market for healthcare. Our only hope is to keep it local and build on what we've got, rather than selling off NHS services to overseas corporations. If Labour had developed fundholding, allowing GP practices to pool their budgets and develop partnerships with managers, hospital staff, IT experts, social services, local businesses and charities, it would have been a far faster route to the integrated, localised, safer NHS that we're still grasping at.

The Bristol scandal, and much of Shipman, happened on the Tories' watch. But it was left to Labour to decide how to deal with the fallout. Would they see it as an opportunity to embrace quality and safety in the NHS? Or would they use it as a stick to beat and control doctors, and drive through their secret privatisation agenda?

FRANK DOBSON
May 1997–October 1999

Dobson was a surprise replacement for Chris Smith, who was publicly against the private finance initiative and made a rash pledge to save Bart's Hospital. Dobson was hardly 'new' Labour, promising to abolish the internal market but then not being allowed to. Gordon Brown did, however, honour his commitment to stick to Tory spending plans, and so much of Dobson's term of office was taken up with fire-fighting stories of scandalous waits and lack of resources.

Dobson was committed to improving quality and reducing inequality, and was persuaded by lobbying parents to hold a public inquiry into the Bristol heart scandal (but not until after the GMC had tried to save its skin first). Dobson generally got on well with everyone, until he took his shoes off. But he pissed off a few doctors by saying on *Newsnight* that he wouldn't let Janardan Dhasmana, the Bristol heart surgeon suspended from operating on children, operate on him. Blair saw him as a night watchman, to lull the electorate and Old Labour into a false sense of security before unleashing Alan Milburn.

Dobson was set up to fail, sent in to bat for the NHS without a helmet, box or pads. Or a bat. With no extra money, he just had to take the flak for the 'epidemic of hospitals short of beds, doctors hunting for beds and patients turned away' that he'd railed about in opposition. Dobson has since found a second wind as backbench opposition to the commercialisation of the NHS, where he speaks with passion and zeal but very little influence.

PRIVATE EYE
Misinformed Consent

20 June 1997

A study of unsupervised surgical training published in the *British Medical Journal*[1] has confirmed what many doctors, and very few patients, suspect: two-thirds of all operations performed by surgeons-in-training are unassisted. Senior house officers are left alone to do their first salivary-gland excisions, hernia repairs and stomach, spleen and gall bladder removals with senior 'support' not even present in the hospital. One rung up the ladder, surgical registrars are doing complex and life-threatening surgery of the liver, gall bladder and pancreas, often in emergency situations. Emergency bowel resections, leaking aortic aneurysms and kidney transplants are all done for the first time unsupervised. The list for head-and-neck surgeons is so unsettling as to be almost unprintable (e.g. radical neck dissection), and even consultants had to perform operations they hadn't witnessed before.

The analysis of all this has focused on the shambles of medical training, brought about by a combination of professional arrogance, dereliction of duty and, most pertinently, because we have fewer doctors per head of population than most other countries in Western Europe. As one consultant put it: 'If every surgeon had to prove competence prior to performing any procedure, the NHS would collapse overnight.'

Another conclusion is that many operations performed in the UK could be subject to legal action. Doctors have a duty to gain informed consent from patients prior to any procedure. According to the GMC: 'every patient has the right to make his or her own decision regarding medical treatment and care, and

[1] *British Medical Journal* 21 June 1997.

in order to make that decision is entitled to have full information regarding the material risks.' What risk could be more material than a junior surgeon performing your major operation for the first time unsupervised? And yet, NHS patients are seldom given information as to the identity of their surgeon, and never whether he or she has proven competence for the operation.

Informed consent has always been a myth. Often consent is left to the junior house officer, who may not have seen or heard of the operation. As a house officer, I consented someone for a choledochoduodenostomy and I'm still not sure what it is. The GMC suggests that patients should only be consented for operations by someone who is competent to perform it. It would help if the person performing the operation could prove his or her competence too, or at least be closely supervised by someone who could. Alas, neither of these goals is achievable with the current level of staffing in the NHS. Some surgeons argue that most trainees performing solo operations for the first time achieve satisfactory results, and that should be enough to reassure the public. However, far too many cock-ups still occur and, for the relatives left behind, discovering the truth is a painful and prolonged business.

If doctors are to continue with the responsibility of regulating themselves, then the least they could do is follow the American example, where surgeons publish audits of their work that are freely available to the public. A few fiddle their figures to make it look like they're doing harder operations (thus making their results appear better than expected) but generally it works well. For trainee surgeons, figures can be grouped with the consultants who are responsible for their training.

Some surgeons argue that British people are too dim to interpret the results and incapable of making allowances for variations in case-mix between surgeons. Those who only operate on low-risk patients will, almost invariably, achieve better results than those who include high-risk (i.e. very unwell) patients. However, it is quite possible to produce two columns of, say, mortality figures, one which lists the predicted mortality for a particular operation based on the case-mix and average UK results, and another that lists the actual mortality of a particular surgical team. And it doesn't take a genius to spot a team that is way below average.

If surgeons are as competent as they would have us believe, then they have nothing to fear from public audit. If not, then health secretary Frank Dobson will have to find a lot more money for surgical training.

Waiting for Sight

15 August 1997
In the last week, I've seen two patients waiting over eighteen months for cataract operations. Their vision has now deteriorated to such an extent that one is effectively housebound and the other regularly scalds herself with the kettle and is covered in bruises from multiple falls. The operation they both require is extremely successful and quick. It can be done as a day case and is therefore not affected by bed blocking from the increase in emergency admissions. The NHS hospital they have been referred to has a full quota of eye surgeons and offers private cataract operations with a nine-day wait. Those who can't afford to pay are waiting seventy-times as long to be treated in the same NHS hospital by the same surgeon using the same equipment. Frank Dobson's pledge to end two-tierism in the NHS is already looking mighty thin.

Labour may blame the previous Government for inheriting the largest ever rise in waiting lists (up 13%, with 47,000 waiting over a year), but it has also inherited an NHS with more money and more surgeons than ever before. The problem lies in what the surgeons actually do. In 1995 the Audit Commission discovered that an average full-time NHS surgeon does just 3–6 hours at an NHS operating table per week. This compares with 20 hours a week in most other EU countries. Indeed, if NHS surgeons operated on NHS patients for just fifteen hours a week, then no-one would have to wait more than six days for an operation. The NHS would become just as fast and remain a lot safer and cheaper than the private sector, removing the need for the current, grossly iniquitous system. So why hasn't it?

Many surgeons are desperate to be given more NHS operating time, as witnessed by the number who put in extra hours in aid of the Conservatives' waiting-list initiative. Outrageous waits of six years or more have all but disappeared, and the 250,000 patients waiting more than a year for surgery in 1989 were reduced to 4,756 by September 1996. Some surgeons claimed that this political expediency had allowed those waiting longer for routine operations to leapfrog over those waiting a shorter time for urgent surgery, but there is little hard evidence for this. The average NHS wait during this time rose slightly from 34 to 42 days, but the scheme was a temporary success. Alas, when the Conservatives stood back and fed the NHS to the internal market, the log-jam quickly reappeared.

Surgeons themselves are not without blame. They control the waiting lists and those with a keen interest in private practice are less enthusiastic about reducing NHS waits. NHS surgeons at present only have to work a maximum of 3.5 days a week, leaving them plenty of time to pursue other interests. The private system in the UK allows insurance companies to write policies that cherry-pick easy acute cases in healthier people, leaving the NHS to provide for the chronic, difficult cases and the very sick. In addition, the NHS has for years acted as a free safety net to bail out private hospital disasters. The response has been not to improve the free service so as to make private care unnecessary, but to invest in additional NHS pay-beds to try to undercut private hospitals.

At present, the NHS employs a large number of consultant surgeons at £50–£70,000 a year (plus pension and perks), who are given the ridiculous operating resources of half a day a week. Teaching, research and administration take up more time, and outpatient clinics can be one never-ending cattle market. But there's also some paid thumb-twiddling and absconding to private competitors. A better solution for surgeons who want to commit to the NHS would be to offer them full operating and audit facilities throughout the year, and pay them to be genuinely full-time (i.e. no private work). Their work could then be targeted at areas of greatest need – like giving old people the gift of sight.

Still Waiting

29 August 1997

My views on waiting lists provoked a balanced response from the medical hierarchy. The suggestion that NHS surgeons are not used in the most efficient way and that some favour private work over NHS commitments was dismissed as 'nonsense' and 'rubbish' by Dr Peter Hawker, deputy chairman of the BMA's Central Consultants and Specialists Committee: 'Everyone knows that the problem is funding.' Even a spokesman from the Royal College of Surgeons was nudged into a response: 'These are unsubstantiated claims . . .'.

Whilst underfunding is clearly the biggest problem facing the NHS, the claim that private practice is detrimental to the NHS is hardly unsubstantiated. In 1995, Dr John Yates of Birmingham University published *Private Eye, Heart and Hip,* which cited clear evidence that waiting list reductions in the UK have in part been hampered by some consultants spending an inappropriate amount of time with private patients. The response from the BMA was predictable – one representative made a vitriolic personal attack on Yates's motives and political views in a radio interview – but the response from grass-roots surgeons was divided. One wrote of his embarrassment at the failure of the profession to tackle abuses, another – on a maximum part-time NHS contract – boasted that four-fifths of his operating was private.

Protectors of the private faith have always argued that it benefits the NHS – that patients who pay for treatment aren't added to NHS lists – but Yates's research in Birmingham showed that consultants cannot be in two places at once and when they try to serve two masters, it is the NHS that suffers. Not that this evidence was easy to come by. He was repeatedly thwarted in his attempts to discover the truth but, with the help of observation by private detectives, managed to compile a formidably detailed dossier of the detrimental effect of private medicine on NHS waits.

Did it do any good? When he presented *prima facie* evidence of abuse at a Birmingham hospital to the regional health authority, they distorted it so much as to conclude no problem existed. The Conservative Government decided to gloss over it too, leaving an angry but persistent Dr Yates searching for more evidence to encourage the NHS to change. He has been joined by Professor Donald Light from Manchester University, who wrote in 12 July's *BMJ*: 'The (current) arrangement provides strong incentives to minimise (i.e. ration) operations for NHS patients and use the NHS as an operating base for maximising private work ... I have been told by consultants that some surgeons walk out with NHS X-rays for their private patients under their arm. This is stealing. If a cook walked out with a ham, she or he would be arrested. Some surgeons work out deals with GPs to take care of their NHS patients promptly, if the GPs will steer patients who can pay over to their private practice. Some surgeons are said to manipulate their waiting lists and what they tell a given patient in order to get patients with money to go private. I am told the distorting effect of these "sweetheart" contracts lead the minority who exploit them to believe that politicians and NHS patients should feel grateful for whatever work they do for the NHS.'

The abusers are very much in the minority and it is far more common to find that NHS surgeons work for more hours than they are paid for. However, for the BMA and Royal College of Surgeons to pretend that none of their flock work the system for pecuniary incentives truly is nonsense, rubbish and unsubstantiated.

Addicted Doctors

19 December 1997

Spare a thought this Christmas for addicted doctors. There are thirteen thousand of us in the UK still practising the noble art whilst dependent on alcohol or drugs – an unbelievable statistic if it didn't come from the British Medical Association (BMA). The BMA is trying to tackle the problem through a 24-hour stress line launched in April 1996. In the first year, 3,300 calls were received, 57% from women doctors, who make up a third of the workforce. A third of the calls dealt with emotional problems (anxiety, stress, depression), a quarter complained about work practices, but very few admitted to an addiction problem. And even fewer were prepared to whistle-blow on a colleague.

The ability of doctors to hide their addictions stems from a combination of intelligence, professional status, peer loyalty and lack of insight. Those who are aware they have a problem are also mindful of coming forward because, according to Dr Clive Froggat, 'there is no effective support system available. Your whole livelihood is threatened and there is little effort put into rehabilitation. So an awful lot of sick doctors are just allowed to practise by their colleagues.'

Froggat has been very public about his addiction since he was exposed in 1995. He started with cannabis as a medical student and progressed to cocaine and heroin in 1989. He got the former on the black market and the latter out of his bag, and for years hid the problem from his wife and partners until a Cheltenham pharmacist became 'deeply suspicious' about his prescribing habits. A month later, there was a very public dawn raid on his house.

Dr Ian Joiner is a recovering alcoholic who still practises as a GP. He has a drinking history spanning 35 years from medical school, peaking at four bottles of gin a week and four drink-driving offences. Dr Joiner was placed under psychiatric supervision for seven years by the GMC and now runs the Addicted Physicians Programme from his front room in Farnham, Surrey: 'Recently I spoke to a cardiac surgeon who was drinking half a bottle of vodka a day so he could steady his hands before an operation. He was unable to take my advice and he's still out there.'

Dr Joiner set up his service in 1995, funded entirely by donations from users, because he was disillusioned by the help offered by the medical establishment. The occupational health service in the NHS is scandalously poor, and it's left to a patchy 'three wise men' procedure in hospital and on Local Medical Committees to sort out problem doctors and protect the public. The National Counselling Service for Sick Doctors offers an informal route to psychiatric services which, in the current climate of the NHS, often fail to provide the necessary supervision to rehabilitate doctors.

The General Medical Council has ultimate responsibility to

protect patients but currently just 140 out of the 13,000 addicts are practising under the GMC's supervision. The GMC's view is that, whilst recognising that it only sees the tip of the iceberg, the local procedures work well to sort out addicted doctors and it's not something the public should worry about. Clive Froggat takes a different view: 'If there are 13,000 addicted doctors making 2,000 vital clinical decisions each year, that's 26 million vital decisions each year made by addicts.' Cheers!

It's hard to find evidence of wholesale patient harm at the hands of addicted doctors, largely because no-one picks up doctors' mistakes. Earlier this year, a fatal-accident inquiry at which it was alleged a consultant surgeon operated under the influence of alcohol led to calls to breathalyse surgeons. Pilots and train drivers have to do it, and doctors may follow suit.

The BMA has set up an action group in Scotland for problem drinkers, but seems to have conceded that what's needed – a humane working environment and a good occupational health service – may never happen. Last month, the BMA gave a huge vote of confidence to the NHS by sending its members details of BUPA personal healthcare with preferential discounts. So now we can all get pissed in private. Merry Christmas.

Pain Special

30 December 1997

If you had crippling pain following an illness, operation or accident, you might expect someone to sort it out. Soon. Certainly, we have the knowledge and the technology. As Dr Douglas Justins, a consultant anaesthetist and pain-management specialist at London's St Thomas's Hospital puts it: 'It's 151 years since the first anaesthetic was given in Britain and in this day and age it's totally unacceptable for anyone still to be suffering acute pain anywhere in a hospital.' Alas, an Audit Commission Report, *Anaesthesia under Examination*, has found that only 57% of hospitals have acute pain-control teams which have been proven to reduce and often eliminate suffering, and that the amount of pain you suffer can depend on which hospital the ambulance drops you off at.

All this prompted Leo Strunin, president of the Royal College of Anaesthetists and a consultant at the Royal London Hospital, to accuse NHS trusts of failing to take patients' suffering seriously: 'Many do not see it as a quality issue. The funds and leadership just aren't there to provide proper pain relief in hospital.' How comforting.

Earlier last year, another report found that children, from neonates on special care upwards, suffered unnecessary pain and that new approaches such as needle-free analgesia, aren't filtering through. In adults, half of all cancer patients and a third of cardiac patients suffer unnecessary pain. Although there has been a 41% increase in the number of consultant anaesthetists over the last ten years, this has been well outstripped by demand and 13% of posts are vacant. Many trusts have barely enough anaesthetists to put people to sleep, let alone administer epidurals to labouring women or run pain clinics.

At undergraduate level, training in pain management is often pitiful, and many health professionals qualify with quaintly stoical views about pain and a reticence to use opioid pain-killers. Morphine is a brilliant painkiller and has been used for centuries, and yet many doctors either refuse to give it or don't give enough for fear of overdosing or causing addiction. 'The reluctance to prescribe morphine is a long-standing problem based on tradition, misconceptions, misinformation and a lack of education,' says Justins. 'It is perceived as a very dangerous drug.' In fact, even when patients are on large doses to control their pain, the chances of becoming a drug addict are 'infinitesimally small.' Over time, the body does become tolerant to the drug and larger doses are needed, but these don't result in overdose. It's far more likely for pain to kick in because a doctor is reluctant to increase the dose.

The best pain relief we have remains misunderstood and underused, as roofer Rod Buck can testify: 'I fell 30 feet off a roof and landed on my back. I broke most of my ribs and the broken ends penetrated the lungs. ... In intensive care, the pain was overwhelming. It was out of this world, it actually paralysed you, you couldn't move, all your muscles clamped up and you were absolutely frozen rigid.'

After two weeks of pain and much forceful complaining, Rod got what he needed: 'I was rescued by an anaesthetic consultant who had a special interest in pain management and prescribed morphine for me. But once I got on the general wards, I was aware of a subtle disapproval on the part of many of the staff of me being on morphine, rather as if I was a sort of an alcoholic or child molester, certainly a person of weak moral fibre, because I was needing to take this stuff.

'I think my experience was unusual because I demanded and got adequate analgesia. I think a lot of people give up in the face of determined opposition of the nursing and junior medical staff.'

Take a tip from Rod. If you suffer excruciating pain in 1998, ask for some morphine. And a pain specialist. Happy New Year.

Cervical Screening is Hard

12 February 1998

The cervical screening fiasco in Kent and Canterbury (eight women dead and 250,000 smears to be rechecked) may not be the only one. The interpretation of slides of cervical smears is not clear-cut or simple, and a decade ago standards were not in place in many labs where poorly paid, overworked screeners had five minutes to interpret what were often very complex cell patterns. As a result, there are potentially twenty or more labs around the country where, if you rigorously examined the work they were doing eight or ten years ago, it would be no different from Kent and Canterbury.

Given the current level of media and legal interest in this topic, it is likely that these centres will be exposed over the next few years. Although surgeons can bury their mistakes, pathologists (and radiologists) leave concrete records of each test, which years later can be given to an expert with hours to spend, knowing that the patient subsequently developed a problem.

Screeners remain overworked and under enormous time pressure today, but all labs now operate double-checks and use safety-net procedures, and overall the incidence of cervical cancer deaths has fallen. Many people mistakenly believe that with immaculate screening, cervical cancer can be eradicated completely. This has never been true, given the unpredictability of some forms of the cancer. For every cancer detected, one will escape detection even with the best screening.

A far greater problem is that just as most labs are getting it right, the adverse press from the consequences of yesterday's low standards is making it extremely difficult to recruit high-quality technicians. Mr Dobson may throw money at the problem but if no-one wants to do the job, the screening programme will be stuffed. Then see what happens to cervical cancer rates.

Cleft Lip and Palate Surgery

26 February 1998

Last November on *Trust Me, I'm a Doctor* (BBC2), I exposed the dismal state of cleft lip and palate repair in the UK, with large numbers of centres doing relatively few operations with poor cosmetic results. A North West of England audit had found that 48% of children require major and often multiple reconstructive surgery, Royal College of Surgeons guidelines were being flouted, and a petty turf war was being fought out by plastic surgeons and maxillo-facial surgeons to the detriment of patients. Now, four months later, the Clinical Standards Advisory Group (CSAG) of the Department of Health has agreed.

After investigating 297 children aged five, and 277 aged twelve, who had all undergone cleft repair in Britain, they found that 40% had poor dental bite, less than a third had a good lip appearance at the age of twelve and under half could speak with normal intelligibility at that age. The CSAG stated that of the 57 centres carrying out the operation, only six to eight provided good-to-excellent care and the overall results were five to twelve times poorer than in the six European centres examined. And the key factors causing poor training and poor results were 'specialists' doing only one or two operations a year and 'competition between plastic and maxillo-facial surgeons'.

It is now almost six years since the *Eye* published the equally unimpressive audit figures for paediatric cardiac surgery at the Bristol Royal Infirmary and highlighted the need for surgical teams not just to audit their work but to act on the results, retiring gracefully from operations which may be beyond them. This latest report found that not only are many surgeons continuing to perform operations they are not competent to do, but they are failing to keep adequate records or perform proper audit.

Only in the area of alveolar bone grafting is there enough information to compare the two specialties and the results are not pretty. 50% of cases carried out by plastic surgeons failed, compared to 32% done by maxillo-facial surgeons. A further factor in this gross incompetence was the desire of hospital managers to keep operations in-house and cheap rather than refer to a more expensive super-specialist centre which may do 50 successful operations a year using highly trained teams.

The false economy and inhumanity of the former approach is illustrated by Dr Symon Whyte, an anaesthetist who had to undergo nine major corrective operations in his childhood because the first repair was not done properly. One operation stuck in his mind: 'It involved breaking the upper jaw on both sides, advancing the jaw so that the bite came into a normal line, taking some bone from my left hip, and grafting that into the gap they'd created in the fracture site. They then welded the whole lot into place with plates so that it was fixed and rigid and the bones could grow together again.' Seven hours in theatre, 24 hours in intensive care, wires and tubes everywhere . . .

Viagra etc.

6 May 1998
British men itching to get their hands on Viagra (sildenafil) – the impotence pill not yet available on the NHS – are trying their luck in Harley Street. However, they should be very wary of the mark-up. Some private clinics have an abysmal record of ripping desperate men off, and prey on the assumption that they will be too embarrassed to question the fee. Many sufferers prefer to answer anonymous private ads in the press than confront their GP – whose knowledge and attitudes may in any case be unhelpful. An Impotence Association Survey found that

half of those men who do see a GP come away dissatisfied and 23% get no treatment at all.

If they do, the commonest prescribed impotence drug in the UK is Caverject (alprostadil), which works in a similar manner to Viagra by relaxing smooth muscle and increasing penile blood flow – but has to be given as a shot in the shaft (not too painful though, I'm told). Alas, impotent men who decide to go private commonly end up paying over £1,000 for a short consultation (worth £60), a few blood tests (worth £100 at most), a trial intra-penile injection of Caverject (£7) and, if it works, a few doses to be getting along with (£30).

A much better and cheaper impotence service is available in parts of the NHS, but you may have to persevere to find it. Some GPs are happy to initiate treatment but others prefer to refer to a hospital clinic, usually run by a urologist or a specialist nurse. Caverject is available on the NHS or, if you prefer, the same drug can be given intra-urethrally (down the end of the penis) in pellet form. This is amusingly known as MUSE. If either suits, you'll be given a small supply and referred back to your GP, who must then decide how much to shell out for your sex life. There is great variability here. As Sister Nolly Biggins, an impotence specialist at Doncaster Royal Infirmary, puts it: 'The good GPs recognise the distress and marital breakdown that impotence can cause and will prescribe enough of the drug for sex twice a week. But I have known male GPs who'll only dish out enough for once a month. I mean, what do they think their knob's for – stirring the tea?'

Viagra, Caverject and Muse don't work for everyone and are not without side effects. Vacuum pumps have been around for years. They're very effective, and have very few side effects, other than a very cold penis. But for some ludicrous reason they are not available on the NHS. As Sister Biggins explains: 'They're very useful for diabetic men, half of whom become impotent and many don't want to take any more drugs. But because the pumps aren't prescribable, I've had to buy some using charitable donations and share them out amongst the patients.' At £200 each, they're not cheap but they recoup the cost of drug treatment in a few months.

Some men who can't afford them buy cheap penis pump enlargers from sex shops or mail ads. 'They're a disaster,' says Sister Biggins. 'They don't work properly and they usually give you a tight plastic ring to slip over the base of the penis to maintain the erection. Often, the ring's so tight that it won't come off and you have to go to casualty to get it cut off.' You have been warned. Always use a penile ring with handles attached.

Colorectal Cancer

20 May 1998
In 1997, the NHS executive published the research evidence for 'improving outcomes in colorectal cancer'. This is the second biggest cancer killer, causing 17,000 deaths a year in England and Wales. It gets more common with age and often presents with bleeding from the rectum or a change of bowel habit.

The survey found large variations in the methods used and success rates for surgery, and concluded that 'surgery for rectal cancer should be concentrated in the hands of surgeons who can demonstrate good results, particularly in terms of low recurrence rates. Surgeons should monitor their performance by working closely with histopathologists.' But only 5% of them do and the rest really haven't got a clue how they're doing.

Even when a surgeon meticulously audits his work and proves that a new technique can bring substantial benefits, it can take fifteen years for these to become widely used. Bill Heald, a Basingstoke surgeon, has pioneered the technique of total mesorectal excision (TME) which involves meticulous removal of the tissues lying circumferentially around the rectum, rather than the traditional process of removing a tumour longitudinally. Recurrence rates, colostomy usage and death are markedly lower in his patients compared to those elsewhere in the UK, and although no randomised controlled trial has been done, population studies in Scandinavia, Holland and Germany are strongly reinforcing this finding. Heald has revolutionised rectal cancer care outside the UK.

The fact that Heald's genius has been embraced by our European partners but largely ignored in the UK says a lot about the way we practise. Surgical training has not in the past allowed the specialisation to learn new skills such as TME, preferring to produce general surgeons who can do a bit of everything. Some can, but others are getting alarmingly high recurrence rates for the cancer and recurrence nearly always means death.

Back in 1986, Heald published his own recurrence rates of 2–6% compared to the national average of 35%. His colostomy rates are 15%, compared to the average of 45%, and by preserving the nerves of sexual function, his impotence rate is also a third that of those using traditional surgery. Indeed, there is more variability in the outcomes for rectal cancer surgery than for any other cancer, so it's vital you get a specialist team that publishes its results.

Eye Plug

3 July 1998
'The role of non-executive members of healthcare trusts has become an issue; their absence from the Bristol story is remarkable, especially given that stories in the satirical magazine *Private Eye* put the issue on the public agenda (a fact that should surely have alerted everyone that there was enough

dissent among staff to persuade someone to leak information to the press).' So observed Rudolf Klein, professor of social policy at Bath University in the *British Medical Journal* (June 6, 1998, p. 1742).

The baton for sorting out this mess will soon be passed to Professor Ian Kennedy, who is to chair the public inquiry. In the meantime, it's worth pointing out that the new paediatric cardiac surgery team in Bristol have mortality rates lower than the national average. For the first time in six years, I'd allow my own children to be operated on there.

A Surgeon's Lot

17 July 1998
At London's Royal Brompton Hospital, cardiothoracic surgeons are effectively on call 24 hours a day, every day. As one put it: 'The policy here is that if a patient that you operated on develops a problem, you are expected to sort it out even if you aren't officially on duty. So you have to carry a pager with you all the time, and be prepared to come back to theatre.' Quite why the surgeons are so reluctant to sort out each other's complications is unclear – perhaps they don't wish to contaminate each other's league tables – but committing to round-the-clock cover means never touching a drop of alcohol, just in case they're called in. What a life.

Although individual surgeons will not be identified when Frank Dobson publishes the rates of post-operative death and other selected complications, surgical units will be named and consultants are worried that they may be tainted by association. The least they can hope for is that a statistical adjustment is made to favour the units who do the hardest operations on the sickest patients. Poor results will be blamed on the consultants, even if the problem operations are done by junior staff, since they are responsible for the training. As one consultant told me: 'We're resigned to the fact that league tables will be here to stay after Bristol, but a lot of us are worried. Even if they're accurate, everyone has a bad year or a bit of bad luck or a poor batch of junior staff every now and then. In the past, we've managed to sort it out in private – but once it's public, a single blip could stuff your private work for good.'

Aortic Aneurysms and Biliary Atresia

31 July 1998

An aortic aneurysm is an abnormal bulging of the major vessel that carries blood out of the heart. 3% of men over 50 have one, usually without any symptoms, and at least a third of these will go on to rupture. This is bad news. Symptoms include severe abdominal pain, often radiating to the back or groins, and collapse. The emergency surgery involves clamping the aorta above the leak and inserting a Dacron graft. Without treatment, the death rate is 100%. With treatment, the death rate depends on how quickly it is picked up – large ruptures at home have a 90% death rate, in hospital the average survival is 50%.

However, a much better outcome can be achieved by screening. With ultrasound, most of the aneurysms can be picked up and operated on before they rupture. When this policy to screen men over 60 was introduced in Chichester, the death rate from ruptured aneurysms fell to zero (i.e. there weren't any) and the death rate from the elective operations was just 1%. In two-thirds of the cases, the aneurysms might not have ruptured but the pick-up rate was far higher than for, say, cervical screening and comparatively many more lives were saved. And although expensive in terms of the initial outlay for screening and the elective operating, the patients didn't require the prolonged intensive care that those having emergency surgery often need. This can lead to a miserable prolonged death from kidney failure and infection.

After the elective operation, the men are then brought back to the mortality rate of their peers (i.e. they live as long as men who don't have aneurysms), giving them up to twenty years extra of high-quality living. So presumably every major centre around the country is offering screening? Alas no. Men who've worked hard and paid tax all their lives are still thought of as low-priority patients, it seems. The cynical view is that it is much cheaper to let them collapse at home and die. As one consultant put it: 'We're probably losing 6,000 men a year through not screening men over 50. Compare that with cervical screening, where we screen all women aged 20 to 65 and save a thousand lives a year.' Without screening, your best bet for survival is to call an emergency ambulance if you get the above symptoms and go straight to hospital.

At the other end of life, my top tip is to take jaundice in babies seriously. Any baby that is still yellow at two to three weeks needs to be assessed. The cause is usually breast-feeding, but biliary atresia, a congenital malformation that prevents bile drainage, must be excluded. And yes, there's a scandal here too. If children are identified early (within six weeks), often they can have a complex operation called a Kasai procedure that takes up to five hours but can improve drainage through the biliary tract. [cf, p. 94]At best, this can completely obviate the need for a liver transplant or at least postpone it for many years. At worst, it does nothing, other than subject a very young baby to life-threatening surgery.

Because the condition is rare, only 50 such operations are carried out in the UK each year. So you'd think they're all done in two or three highly specialised centres which do enough of the procedures to ensure they're good at them. Unbelievably, there are fifteen centres doing the operation, with many carrying out just one or two a year. King's Hospital London and

Birmingham are the centres of excellence, doing most of the operations and clearly they should be doing them all – their success rates are double those of the dabblers. So if your child is offered this operation at another centre, insist on going to King's or Birmingham. [cf. p. 95]

More Biliary Atresia

27 August 1998

The Kasai operation is a complex procedure used to correct biliary atresia, a congenital malformation that prevents bile drainage, and two factors determine its success: (a) the speed with which the diagnosis is made and (b) the skill of the surgical team. At best, the children remain jaundice-free for many years and may never need a liver transplant. At worst, the operation fails and the baby needs a transplant to survive in the next year or two. So the stakes are high.

Back in 1985, the *British Medical Journal* published a survey of the results of this treatment conducted between 1980 and 1982.[1] Ninety-five children had the Kasai operation. They were treated at sixteen different centres by at least sixteen different surgeons, and success was measured according to whether the children were free of jaundice from 10 months to 3.5 years. Good results were clearly related to the number of cases operated on in each centre. Only 11% of children treated in centres dealing with one case a year were free of jaundice compared with 29% at centres treating two to five cases a year and 45% at King's College Hospital, London – the only centre to treat more than five cases a year.

---

[1] McClement J, Howard E, Mowat A. Results of surgical treatment for extrahepatic biliary atresia in United Kingdom 1980–2. *British Medical Journal* 2 February 1985; 290: 345–7.

The paper deduced that this alarming variability in results was 'probably' down to 'the experience of the surgeon and the standard of care'. It concluded that the outlook for these children would be improved if 'treatment was concentrated in a few centres, in each of which the vast majority of operations are done by one surgeon'. Thirteen years later, you'd imagine it was all sorted out. Dream on. The survey for 1993–95 found that fifteen centres were still doing the Kasai operation and although the overall success rates have improved, the same depressing variability exists.

The average success rates for the two units doing more than five operations a year (King's and Birmingham Children's) is 62%, those doing two to five is 50% and those doing one a year is 17%. Based on this information, I recommended that children should only be referred to King's or Birmingham. This provoked a prompt response from Mark Stringer, a consultant paediatric surgeon at Leeds General Infirmary, whose own figures are comparable to the best. So Leeds can be added to the recommended list, but I wouldn't go to units that do one operation a year. As Mr Stringer puts it: 'We need to prevent surgeons carrying out this operation on rare occasions and the British Association of Paediatric Surgeons has been taking steps to achieve this.' It's now just thirteen years since their last survey proposed to do exactly that. But hey, it's only eight-week-old babies we're dealing with.

And what of the parents? The downfall of the surgeons in Bristol was not their poor performance *per se*, but that they had quoted parents national survival rates for operations when their own figures were far worse. Are parents of children with biliary atresia treated at the 'one a year' centres being told the local success rate is 17%, compared with 62% elsewhere? I suspect not.

On the Nose

11 September 1998

A patient recently turned up to ear, nose and throat outpatients at Southampton University Hospitals NHS trust and was turned away for being a year early. He hadn't spotted that the waiting time for a routine appointment (i.e. the time taken to see a doctor even before you go on the waiting list) is 60 weeks. This is clearly unacceptable, but hardly surprising when you consider that there are more ENT consultants in New York State than the whole of the UK and clinics are already ludicrously busy. One junior ENT surgeon in Leicester regularly sees more than 30 patients in a three-hour outpatient clinic and his record is 44. This works out at four minutes per patient, including turnaround time, when the recommended appointment time for good-quality practice is fifteen minutes. Clinics become cattle markets and everyone ends up dissatisfied.

The obvious solution is to train more junior staff and create more consultant posts for them to go to. Alas, this can meet barriers from managers ('too expensive') and some existing consultants who don't want anyone cutting into their lucrative private work. In Southampton, two of the ENT specialists have vetoed another consultant appointment and opted instead for an associate specialist. Associate specialists cost less than a consultant but very few are accredited for their training, some have repeatedly failed membership or fellowship of their royal college, and the ones I've met are deeply unhappy and disillusioned with their lot. They can never become consultants but they're allowed to do a lot of the consultant's work, usually unsupervised. This is hardly a guarantee of the quality service Frank Dobson bangs on about, and yet the *BMJ* job section is full of adverts for associate specialists.

In the short term, Dobson is trying to solve the problem of long waiting lists by paying consultants private-size fees to operate on NHS patients in private hospitals at weekends. For example, the orthopaedic consultants in Southampton have received £2.5 million to get their lists down. This strategy – also used unsuccessfully by the Tories – comes on the back of a report by the charity Action for Victims of Medical Accidents, which has found that a disproportionate number of the claims it deals with are coming out of the private sector. Key factors are the lack of both emergency equipment and medical expertise. Private hospitals are not the places to be in an emergency.

Blind Amniocentesis

19 November 1998

If you were pregnant, would you let an obstetrician stick a needle into your uterus without knowing where the baby is? It happens every day in the UK. Amniocentesis involves drawing off fluid from around the baby in the womb to diagnose conditions such as Down syndrome. It's usually performed at sixteen weeks and parents are told that the risk of causing miscarriage is between 0.5% and 1%. However, in some hands, the risk may be much higher. An unpublished audit at a centre in Wales found a miscarriage rate of 4%, eight times worse than the best centres. Why?

A successful amniocentesis depends on the needle reaching the amniotic fluid in the womb without hitting the baby. For over fifteen years, ultrasound equipment has allowed continuous monitoring so that the needle tip is always in view during the procedure, as well as the placenta and the baby (which has a habit of moving around). It requires training and considerable skill to operate the ultrasound equipment and guide the needle at the same time and, as you'd expect in a service as patchy as the NHS, some obstetricians (both junior and senior) don't have it. But they do amniocentesis anyway.

How? They do the ultrasound first, find out where the baby is, put the scanner down, pick up the needle and hope that the baby doesn't move. But often it does. And even if you manage to avoid the baby, you may hit the placenta which can have equally catastrophic effects. Bad amniocentesis can not only cause miscarriage, but there's increasing evidence it could also lead to brain damage in surviving infants.

If amniocentesis is done blind, the only way of knowing you're in the right spot is if the syringe is filled with clear amniotic fluid. If it's filled with blood, you've bodged up, but you get rid of it quickly, hope the parents don't notice and have another go. This is clearly unacceptable practice, but it wasn't until 1996 that the Royal College of Obstetricians and Gynaecologists got round to issuing guidelines, stating that amniocentesis must be performed under continuous ultrasound with the tip of the needle always in view.

Alas, Royal Colleges carry very little clout and some obstetricians just carry on doing it the old way. Eric Jauniaux, a foetal medicine expert at University College Hospital, sees a woman a week who has had a failed amniocentesis: 'In most of the cases they tell me that there wasn't any ultrasound guidance at the time of the procedure.'

As with most of medicine, training is poor and there's very little quality control of ultrasound use and amniocentesis in individual centres. So it's very difficult for women to find out whether or not the person performing their amniocentesis is adequately trained and competent. Diane Parnell was unlucky. When she went for her amniocentesis, she was scanned before, but not during, the procedure: 'The gynaecologist came in and looked at the scan picture that had been taken minutes before ... the needle was inserted into my womb and then Terry [her husband] said: "It's failed, he's going to have to do it again." Same problem, same pain if not more, and blood swirling round in the syringe.'

Diane did not miscarry, but her daughter Mishka was born blind and deaf, with severe brain damage. There was a large scar on the scalp, right over where the damage was. Mishka died when she was two. The hospital admitted the amnio was done badly, but they insisted the needle could not have caused Mishka's brain damage. The Parnells turned for help to Oxford pathologist Waney Squier, who has now done a study of brain scans and slides taken from Mishka and other children with similar injuries. She has linked developmental damage precisely to the time of the amniocentesis in each case.

Many obstetricians won't acknowledge the huge variation in miscarriage rates or the brain damage that can result from botched amniocentesis. At present, the only way of ensuring it isn't done blind is for patients themselves to do quality checks on doctors. This is incredibly difficult. A woman who is already petrified she might have a baby with a congenital abnormality, lies on her back and faces an obstetrician with a needle. Is she going to ask if continuous ultrasound guidance is being used? Recently, I was contacted by two women, one from Manchester whose amniocentesis was done blind by a consultant who didn't speak to her and drew blood on two occasions before giving up. But another woman due to have an amniocentesis at the Alexandra Healthcare NHS Trust in Redditch found out the consultant she was offered did it blind and insisted on seeing someone else.

She eventually got good treatment, but only by asserting herself. Most women are frightened of challenging doctors, as the horrific injuries inflicted by Kent gynaecologist Rodney Ledward will testify. He was dubbed 'the Butcher' by his colleagues at William Harvey Hospital in Ashford. They had to repair his cock-ups and yet they didn't stop him operating in the first place. Likewise, the majority of competent obstetricians in this country who are doing amniocentesis properly are aware of those in their department who aren't. But will they stop them? No. As ever, the secretive self-regulation of doctors stinks.

Time to Regulate Perfusionists

19 November 1998

Would you want your life support machine operated by an unregulated technician? Probably not. Yet the perfusionists who operate heart-lung bypass machines during open-heart surgery on babies, children and adults have no regulation at all. This fact hit the press recently after a baby undergoing surgery at Guy's Hospital bled to death in seconds when a heart bypass machine modified by an unsupervised trainee perfusionist suffered a catastrophic failure. Four-month-old Hannah Shepherd died after a tube connecting her to the machine 'blew off and whirled around the room,' covering the floor in blood. Hannah was pronounced dead twenty minutes later.

Describing Hannah's death as 'violent and shocking,' Dr Selena Lynch, the Southwark coroner, called on the Government to urgently consider imposing registration and regulation controls on the operators of heart-lung bypass machines to minimise the chance of it happening again. She is preparing a report to send to the Department of Health (DoH). This plea, however, is old news to the DoH. For some years, perfusionists themselves have applied to become regulated under the Council for the Professions Supplementary to Medicine. A submission in June 1996 was made by the Perfusion Liaison Group of the Society of Perfusionists of Great Britain and Ireland comprising, amongst others Magdi Yacoub, Professor of Cardiac Surgery at the Royal Brompton Hospital and other eminent cardiac surgeons and anaesthetists. It failed. At every stage, obstacles were presented by none other than the Department of Health.

Poor Stroke Services

28 December 1998

What's the single main cause of disability in the UK? What's the third biggest killer? And what's being done about it? Stroke, stroke and not much. Each year 100,000 people suffer a stroke – that's one every five minutes – with often devastating consequences. 5.8% of the entire NHS and social services budget is spent on treatment, and most of that goes on 'rehabilitation'. Fortunately, there is good evidence that patients treated in specialist units do better. Back in 1993, the *Lancet*[1] published an overview of all the randomised controlled trials between 1962 and 1993 comparing specialist stroke management with non-specialist. Patients treated in stroke units were 28% more likely to be alive after four months and 21% more likely to make it to a year. In nine out of ten of the units, the patients also achieved 'functional gains' (i.e. were less disabled after treatment).

In 1997, the *British Medical Journal* published a similar review which found that specialist stroke care reduced the chances of dying or remaining physically dependent by 29%.[2] If all patients had access to such care, over 4,500 lives a year would be saved and another 6,250 patients would regain independence, compared to conventional care. There is no increase in the use of resources with such care and there is some evidence that hospital stays may be shorter. There is also the potential for huge savings in that many thousands of patients would not need long-term institutional care nor draw disability benefits, and the burden on carers, who currently put in 3.7 million hours a week, would be much reduced.

The Department of Health has at least recognised that stroke care is a problem, costing £2.3 billion a year with

[1] *Lancet* 1993; 342: 395–8.
[2] *BMJ* 1997; 314: 1151–9.

patients occupying 20% of acute hospital beds and 25% of long-term beds. The Government's 'Our Healthier Nation' targets include a reduction in the death rate from heart disease and stroke amongst those under 65 by a further third. However, despite a recent report by the Clinical Standards Advisory Group that found widespread variations in stroke treatment and care, the Government has yet to announce any national implementation for organised stroke care. If such a scheme had been implemented in 1993 when the evidence of benefit was clear, many thousands of stroke patients would have been alive and free from disability.

At present, the stroke care you or your relatives receive is a postcode lottery, with those who make it to a specialist unit 29% more likely to survive and regain independence. If there is no such unit in your area, you (or your relatives) should insist on being taken to one.

Private Malpractice

30 January 1999

At present, anyone can call themselves a consultant in cosmetic surgery, open a clinic and perform surgery, provided they don't claim to have a medical degree. And a physiotherapist struck off by his or her regulatory body (the Register of the Council for the Professions Supplementary to Medicine) can open a private clinic that afternoon and practise as a ... er ... physiotherapist. And even though doctors in private practice are within the remit of GMC regulation, very few are called to account for misconduct. Anyone, however slim, can obtain amphetamines for weight loss from doctors in private slimming clinics. And wealthy addicts worried about their next fix can pop off to Harley Street and buy whatever they want. The doctor gains a huge fee for the consultation and the pharmacist gets a huge mark-up on the prescription. All grossly unethical but entirely legal.

Even 'routine' private practice is open to widespread abuse. Because of the pecuniary incentive to investigate or operate, patients may be given unnecessary tests or treatments or, just as alarming, be operated on by surgeons with no expertise in that particular area. In a letter to the *BMJ* (Vol. 317, p. 811 [September 19, 1998]), obstetrician Beverley Webb, chairman of the medical advisory committee at Pinehill Hospital, Hitchin, Hertfordshire wrote:

'Unnecessary operations are a great problem, some being performed by doctors who have had only basic training in the techniques while they were passing though a specialty. . . . What does one do if a colleague who is not an orthopaedic surgeon or hand surgeon operates on Dupytren's contractures, or a colleague who is not a plastic surgeon performs breast reductions, or a colleague who is not a gynaecologist inappropriately operates on genital prolapse? What do you do if a colleague always finds something to operate on no matter what the patient is referred with? And what do you say to the anaesthetist who always puts in a regional block as well as giving a general anaesthetic in order to bump up the fee?

'It astounds me that the medical insurance companies themselves have not policed these sorts of activities in order to reduce their own financial outgoings. All of these examples are observed every week by all of us who have our eyes open. Worse, they are obvious to our nursing and paramedical colleagues, who wonder why we are doing nothing to correct these anomalies . . .' Alas, if a cockup occurs in private practice (and this is increasingly common according to a report by Action for Victims of Medical Accidents), patients don't have recourse to the NHS complaints or compensation procedures.

A Victory for the *Eye*

6 May 1999

Last August, the *Eye* suggested that babies with biliary atresia should be treated at either Birmingham, Leeds or King's, London – the three expert centres treating enough patients to produce statistically meaningful results. Nine months later, Frank Dobson agrees. In a press release from the Department of Health (April 30), the health secretary has agreed with all of the *Eye*'s proposals.

Not everyone is happy. In a letter to the *British Medical Journal*, five consultants from Booth Hall Children's Hospital and Royal Manchester Children's Hospital have complained that the *Eye*'s coverage was 'inaccurate and misleading' (*BMJ*, April 10). Manchester was a 'medium-volume centre' with an average success rate of 54% and, if biliary atresia was a common disease, it might well have been chosen as another specialist centre. However, with only 50 cases a year there is only a need for three such centres. Any more would dilute the expertise and make any audit much less reliable.

The argument that parents want their babies to be treated locally rather than travel further was dismissed by the Children's Liver Disease Foundation. As chief executive Catherine Arkley put it: 'Parents would move to hell and back to get the best for their children.' I have also spoken to the parents of children who had unsuccessful surgery at local non-specialist centres without knowing that such a disparity in results existed. They feel outrage and guilt that this information was not made available to them (when it has been apparent since 1984).

The Manchester team were clearly providing a much better service than those doing just one operation a year and are angry that the debate has been held in the media rather than behind the closed doors of the profession. Consultants at

Birmingham Children's Hospital are also annoyed that their audit was published first in the *Eye* rather than the *Lancet*. Professional journals like to have first bite, and if something has been leaked to the media first, they will often refuse to publish.

However, the information came from concerned doctors working in the field who felt the public-interest element was so strong, it was worth risking a breach of confidentiality and professional censure to get it into the public domain. The latest biliary atresia audit had been sitting on desks since 1996 and, aside from minor statistical adjustments, is as the *Eye* published it. The profession may have eventually got round to weeding out the surgeons who were attempting rare, complex operations on babies and getting demonstrably poor results, but the public exposure of this scandal – admittedly painful for some parents – has had a huge impact on speeding up the process.

As ever, the whistle-blowers must insist on remaining anonymous for fear of reprisals. Little has changed in the seven years since Bristol, except perhaps that the Royal College of Surgeons moves a little quicker. It was the first professional body to act on the biliary atresia audit. However, its president, Barry Jackson, refutes the *Eye*'s claim that the Royal College of Surgeons knows the identity of poorly performing surgeons through its confidential audits. The claim was based on a 1996 interview given by an RCS spokesman, the late Brendan Devlin, who told BBC2's *Trust Me I'm A Doctor* that he was aware of the identity of 'No. 169', a surgeon with very poor results for prostate surgery.

'I can state now – unequivocally – that the college has never known the identity of No. 169,' writes Mr Jackson. 'Brendan Devlin did, as the then director of the Comparative Audit Service, but this was privileged information.' Alas, he's now dead. As for the *Eye*'s other question (what's the point of spending millions on audit if you can't identify the poor performers and prove to the public they've been sorted out?), Mr Jackson has promised to reply shortly in greater detail. In the meantime, No. 169 could still be out there. Look for a tattoo behind the left ear.

ALAN MILBURN
October 1999–June 2003

Alan Milburn, affectionately known as 'Bastard', was in the ideal situation to break a few windows. He had a clutch of medical scandals (Bristol, Shipman, Alder Hey, assorted rogue gynaecologists) to use as evidence to tighten control over doctors, and enough money to sweeten the pill of a market reform programme that was beyond Thatcher's dreams. He was the Marmite health minister – loathed or loved.

Milburn's baptism was one of the worst winters on record, but the bad press included Lord Winston's tirade about his mother's treatment which bounced Blair into announcing that NHS funding would match the European average. He pushed through Labour's NHS Plan on the pretence that it was built around the needs of patients, rather than a veiled invitation to let private competition into the NHS. Doctors didn't spot the deception until too late, because we didn't understand management jargon like 'additionality', 'contestability' and 'introducing diversity into provision'.

Milburn's undoing was his attempt to micromanage the NHS from the centre with impatient haste. He threw so much shit at the walls that some of it had to stick, but as none of his reforms was piloted or evaluated, it's hard to say which bits. Lots of tough targets were set, and lots of figures were fiddled to meet them. Thanks to the Bristol Inquiry report, Milburn introduced standards, inspections and some measure of quality control into the NHS, but it was aggressively, centrally imposed. Many doctors saw him as a bully and he struggled to get them onside, which could be one reason why he suddenly gave up to spend more time at home. The lesson? You can't run the NHS or a family from Whitehall. And doctors want time for their children too.

PRIVATE EYE
Accepting the Buck

21 October 1999

Frank Dobson's swift and unseemly departure from the Department of Health was not only, it seems, to spike Ken Livingstone's mayoral ambitions. Prime Minister Blair's dream of unleashing a radical health agenda on the 'dark forces of Conservatism' (i.e. the BMA) would not have sat well with Dobson's Old Labour beliefs. So enter Alan 'Modernisation is here to stay' Milburn, whose recent stint as health minister led to him being branded 'anti-doctor' by Professor John Ward, vice-president of the Royal College of Physicians. The BMA's Dr Peter Hawker invited him to 'stop attacking the profession and defend doctors' performance.' Mr Milburn took no notice at all and, now he's in charge, he'll take on the medical profession in ways that Margaret Thatcher wouldn't have dared. But is he prepared to take ultimate responsibility for the quality of care in the NHS?

The *Eye*'s repeated exposure of surgical scandals has shown how reluctant the Department of Health has been to accept responsibility without the agreement of the Royal Colleges, which are deeply self-protective and self-serving. If Milburn tries to wrestle control away from the medical profession, he can be sure his civil servants will not be lining up behind him to accept it. And the General Medical Council only launches itself into action years after the event, to save its skin. The GMC gets away with it because no-one else wants to take on responsibility for regulating doctors, especially when most of our cock-ups are tied up with lack of manpower, training and resources. As Mr Milburn will soon find out, you get the health service you pay for and the doctors you deserve.

A good start would be to collect, learn from and publish outcomes so at least we know what we're dealing with. Recently, the Audit Commission published *Critical to Success*, a report into the quality of care in intensive care units in England and Wales. Death rates vary greatly, with some units having thrice the average mortality. Do we know the good ones? Do we know the bad ones? Do we have any guarantee that the bad ones will be sorted out? Do we buggery. It had to be kept a secret 'to encourage units to participate'. So much for freedom of information.

Who Picks Up Doctors' Mistakes?

18 November 1999
Can you make the NHS safer from the top down? We now have a National Institute for Clinical Excellence (NICE) to sift through the evidence and decide on what the NHS should (and shouldn't) provide, and the Commission for Health Improvement, to ensure that NICE's diktats are observed. The commission's first job has been to change its acronym from CHIMP (the ape-association was deemed too flippant) to CHI (half a celebrity panda).

Whether either of these quangos will change behaviour on the ground is debatable. For over ten years Dr William Pickering, a GP with wide experience of medico-legal work, has campaigned for an independent medical inspectorate by asking 'who picks up doctors' mistakes?' Pickering has concentrated on the very basic and rudimentary clinical errors that any reasonably competent doctor should avoid. These generally involve the unnecessarily late diagnosis of treatable disease and the improper supervision of ongoing medical treatment.

In his medico-legal work, Pickering has seen repeated examples of doctors of all ages and ranks failing to follow basic medical rules. For example, failing to investigate blood in the urine resulting in death from undiagnosed bladder cancer or failure to put a patient with a heart attack or a stroke on medication to prevent a further attack. Errors such as these happen every day in the NHS but even when they result in patient harm, they are rarely picked up or commented on. Even at the simplest of levels, there is no systematic way of identifying and acting on doctors' individual mistakes.

Pickering believes that an independent medical inspectorate, headed by doctors with a presence in every region, would be a huge step forward. Only doctors have the easy access to patient records necessary to make an informed judgement, and they have a much clearer idea of what is acceptable practice. The inspectors would not, however, be employed by the NHS and would therefore be less likely to let misguided loyalty get in the way of rational thought. Just an idea.

Gagging for a Lord

10 January 2000
This year's NHS winter crisis had the added spice of Lord Winston's diatribe in the *New Statesman* about how we spend even less of our GDP on health than Poland. This after his mother fell, unobserved, out of an NHS bed. Tony Blair's response has been to bully the good Lord into a retraction, perhaps with the threat of a complaint to the GMC (for divulging that heavily pregnant Cherie has decided not to push and pant). But Winston at least panicked Blair into promising to raise NHS funding to European levels.

Winston need not have retracted. Any genuine concern he raises about the NHS should be protected by the Public Interest

Disclosure Act, which became law last July to prevent the persecution of whistle-blowers. And everyone knows Cherie Blair had a caesarean section last time round and so is highly likely to have another given her age. They might even shave a little of her pubic hair off prior to the incision. This amounts to nothing more than informed speculation and – given that Winston is not in any way involved in her medical care – this does not constitute a breach of confidentiality.

Alas, politicians suffused with self-importance seem incapable of making this distinction. In July 1998, Gregor Mackay – then press secretary to William Hague – reported me directly to the GMC for disrespectful speculation about the Leader of the Opposition's prolonged absence from work: 'I thought the article highly unprofessional and a poor advert for your profession,' fumed Mackay, who was sacked shortly afterwards. After due consideration, the GMC concluded that as I have never been Mr Hague's doctor, my comments were of no interest to them. Ditto Lord Winston and Cherie. Even if she's having it on all fours in Lord Archer's Jacuzzi.

Fortunately, nurses seem less inclined than Lord Winston to be gagged. As community nurse Barbara Mathews from Swansea writes in the *Nursing Times*: 'I am frequently appalled by the basic lack of nursing care for some of my older patients in hospital. They develop painful pressure sores that take months to heal. Drinks are placed out of reach, false teeth not cleaned, food left untouched. I know staff levels are low, but they always were.'

And that's the point. This winter has been no different from every winter in the NHS, in terms of the level of sickness. However, many NHS staff swallowed Labour's trite 'things can only get better' line and believed that, a few years into office, they genuinely would. The fact that so little has changed in the NHS has led to widespread disillusionment, with a knock-on effect on patient care. Lord Winston is just the tip of a very angry iceberg.

TRUST ME, I'M (STILL) A DOCTOR

Trust Me, I'm Still A Doctor

3 February 2000

Harold Shipman is free to doctor his fellow prisoners, despite his fifteen murder convictions, since the GMC is prohibited from taking action while a criminal investigation proceeds, and will be further delayed if Shipman appeals. Once criminal proceedings are completed, the GMC is then required to give 28 days' notice of the intention to suspend a doctor from the register. So Shipman can call himself a doctor for some while yet.

Many doctors now have little faith in the GMC's ability to regulate the profession. As Dr Bill Pickering writes: 'One important reason that Shipman got away with it for so long was because he knew that in the NHS, and in general practice in particular, doctors can do more or less what they like. They call it "clinical freedom" and cherish it. No one (except the law) can meaningfully challenge their actions, and then only if they are found out. Medical ethics do not include commenting on another doctor's practice, nor do they insist upon an open mentality. The "self-regulation" of doctors is, therefore, equivalent to no regulation.'

Unaffordable Drugs

17 February 2000

Last July, the board of the Royal Surrey Hospital NHS Trust asked their solicitors for advice on behalf of consultants who were unable to prescribe expensive drugs for the treatment of ovarian cancer because their budget for such treatments had been cut by £150,000. The consultants wanted to know whether they should tell patients the truth: 'There is a drug that might help you but we can't afford it.' Or whether to resort to kind but dishonest paternalism: 'There is no effective treatment for you.'

The Trust could have afforded the drug eighteen months previously, but is now £1.4 million in the red. As Professor Hilary Thomas, a cancer specialist, put it: 'I have patients who are young and relatively fit and I have a dilemma about whether I am completely honest with them and leave them with the awful thought that if they were private patients, they would be offered the drug.' The Trust's solicitors advised that doctors should always be entirely open and honest with patients, even if it leaves Prof. Thomas with some tough consultations. One patient of his was denied the drug (Hycamtin or topotecan) and died shortly afterwards. He then had to face her husband knowing she hadn't been given the best possible chance of living.

Elsewhere, the information given to patients about ovarian cancer drugs still varies widely between consultants. As a Bristol cancer specialist told me last week: 'One consultant won't mention the ovarian cancer drugs at all if there is no funding for them, because it's cruel. In effect, you're saying, "There is a drug that may help you and it is available in some parts of the NHS but not this one, so tough." The second consultant tells patients these drugs exist to allow the rich ones to buy them privately and the poor ones to go to the papers and try to raise the money in a campaign (which is usually too late to be successful). And the third consultant tells patients that they can't have the drugs and they should lobby their MPs.'

If patients have a right to information about effective treatments their health authority won't pay for, do they also have a right to know about centres of excellence their health authority won't send them to? A recurring problem the *Eye* has repeatedly exposed is that non-specialist units which lack the expertise and resources to do complex procedures continue to do so, and are effectively protected from accountability because the numbers of patients they treat are so small as to be statistically meaningless. But what if a surgeon was obliged to say: 'I only do a couple of these a year, my results mean nothing but I'd like to have a go anyway. And by the way, there's a specialist centre a hundred miles away where they do lots of these, have all the resources and specialist staff and get statistically good results. But you can't go there.'

A few operations are designated to specialist centres, which should guarantee funding, and the Government also has a scheme to allow health authorities to fund treatments outside their area with the catchy title of OATS (out-of-area treatment scheme). However, this is, according to a DoH release, intended primarily for emergencies and like everything else in the NHS is severely cash-limited. This rationing, according to Oxford neurosurgeon Tipu Azis, is sowing the seeds for another Bristol: 'For more complex operations, local units are unlikely to ever develop the critical mass of competence that specialist centres have. As in Bristol, there is a very real risk that a relatively inexperienced team could produce unacceptable results.

'Some procedures are done locally two or three times a year, when I do them two or three times a week. The Government is hypocritical in that it criticised the Bristol heart surgeons yet it is encouraging the same situation to occur in multiple specialties across the country.' Mr Azis, a Labour supporter, has every reason to be angry. In the last few years, referrals to his unit for the treatment of the tremors of Parkinson's disease have plummeted, even though he openly audits his work and has an 80% success rate. His fear is that either patients are not getting the treatment they need – or they may be getting it done badly. Either way, it would be much cheaper to the NHS in the long-term to pay for treatment to be done properly in specialist centres first time round.

Penis Dabbling

6 April 2000

In the NHS you can't always have the very best but you at least deserve to avoid the bodgers. Especially when someone's cutting open your penis. Hypospadius is a common condition, affecting around 1% of boys in the UK, and occurs when the urethra doesn't make it to the end of the penis, but opens on the underside. In the right hands, a two-stage operation will restore a perfect functioning penis. In the wrong hands, you end up with something that looks like the butcher's dog has eaten it and sprays urine all over the place. You have to sit down to pee but, being embarrassed and not knowing any alternative options, you grow up accepting this and never have sex.

Aivar Bracka, a plastic surgeon in Stourbridge, specialises in genital reconstruction operations, gets excellent results and has the audit (and photographs) to prove it. His hypospadius operations are a work of art, but about a third of them are 'salvage procedures' – trying to put right the damage done by previous surgery. He showed me a shocking photo of a man who'd had 50 failed operations on his penis. Why did he keep going back? He was ashamed and embarrassed, he wasn't offered another opinion and the hospital staff kept telling him his surgeon was 'a lovely man' and he was in 'good hands'.

In the present system, there's nothing to stop any urologist, paediatric surgeon or general surgeon having a go at once-a-year hypospadius surgery. But as patients or parents very rarely shout the results from the rooftops, the damage is usually kept under wraps. At the age of four, identical twins Henry and Charlie Phipps had failed surgery at a non-specialist centre. They were both in extreme pain after the operation, and Charlie had to be rushed back to theatre to be catheterised – only they didn't have the right-sized catheter so they used a feeding tube. And when he finally came to 'try out his new willy', the urine came out of five holes like a colander. Henry had a similar result.

Sue and Peter Phipps decided to decline the offer of more surgery and went in search of a specialist, ending up with Bracka, who performed a miraculous transformation. But Jake Marshall went under the knife four times before he got to see a specialist. As his mother Sarah put it: 'I just can't describe the feeling that your son's been butchered by somebody. And he shouldn't be allowed to do it.' Fair point.

Whitewash of the Week

The Ritchie Report into the gynaecological devastation caused by Rodney 'The Butcher' Ledward is the usual old bollocks. Something must be done . . . lessons will be learned . . . blah de blah de blah. The failings have been loosely directed at managers, but none have been called to account, disciplined or asked to go on retraining. Why did the health authority not act, having paid out for Ledward's failed surgery on at least nineteen occasions between 1980 and 1994? Why was he not sacked, rather than allowed to retire and keep his full pension? And how did he become a consultant in the first place?

As a Professor of Obstetrics who worked with Ledward as a junior doctor put it: 'He was a cowboy even then. The worst I've ever come across in my career. Whoever gave him good references and supported his consultant appointment perjured their soul to the devil and will carry their consequences to the grave.' Alas, surgeons do not have to perform a practical at interviews but someone, somewhere must have written Rodney sparkling references. I think we should be told who.

Another GMC Cock-up

11 August 2000

Hot on the heels of Rodney Ledward is rogue gynaecologist Richard 'Struck Off in Canada in 1985 but fit to practise in the UK' Neale. The GMC's defence for not protecting patients from his dreadful surgery is that it is only allowed by law to take the criminal convictions of overseas doctors into account when considering an application to practise in the UK.

Neale was already working in the Friarage Hospital in Northallerton, North Yorkshire when he was erased from the Canadian register. The GMC was informed of this by the Canadian panel, and by Neale's former colleague and friend Dr Andrew Sear: 'The GMC basically told me that what a doctor did in another country was no concern of theirs.'

A string of senior NHS doctors somehow contrived to give Neale excellent references for his clinical care. So why then did the GMC belatedly conclude that he botched scores of operations, left women haemorrhaging, performed surgery without consent and carried out substandard work?

The secretive self-regulation of doctors is still a sham. The Government and GMC have nothing in place to stop another Bristol, Ledward or Neale from recurring. As Richard Neale said in his final plea to the GMC:

'So what am I? A surgeon who had his best interests at heart.'

'Would you read that again please?'

'So what am I? A surgeon who had his best interests at heart . . .'

'Can I just pause? I asked you twice to read the first sentence again. In my copy it says, "A surgeon who had his patients' best interests at heart."'

'What did I say?'

'Your best interests.'

'I beg your pardon, a Freudian slip.'

A Member for Life

29 September 2000

Alan Maynard, director of health policy at the University of York, has written to the *Eye* with his interpretation of how dodgy gynaecologist Richard Neale got away with it for so long: 'It seems that when Northallerton Trust discovered both his awful results in Canada and his incapacity to improve in North Yorkshire, they paid him over £100,000 in 'compensation' and gave him a good reference so he could continue his pain and misery elsewhere. But was NHS management to blame for this?'

Not entirely, argues Maynard, who cites the ridiculous regulations that NHS managers are bound by, and which successive governments have refused to change. At present, a consultant cannot be sacked without 'due cause', and the disciplinary procedure is so protracted that it allows doctors to appeal to the Secretary of State. The doctor may be suspended for years on full pay, leaving no funds for a replacement, while waiting lists rise leaving hospitals facing further penalties for failing to meet government targets. So it's far easier (and cheaper) to let a deviant keep operating.

Maynard also points out that although the GMC is embarrassingly inept at self-regulation, it is the Royal Colleges who are responsible for overseeing training. Ten years ago, when minimally invasive (keyhole) surgery was introduced, training was patchy to non-existent and a great deal of harm was caused by surgeons learning the ropes. And those surgeons found guilty of serious professional misconduct by the GMC (e.g. the Bristol two, Neale, Ledward) don't even have their Royal College affiliations withdrawn. Once a member, always a member – unless you fail to pay the annual subscription (got to keep those wine cellars stocked).

A Day Out in Bristol

18 December 2000

I got a warm welcome when I accompanied a relative for heart surgery at the Bristol Royal Infirmary last month. As one member of staff remarked to the professor of surgery, 'You know who that is, don't you? You'd better not fuck this one up.' Fortunately, the standards of angiography and surgery were superb and any lingering doubts about the expertise of the staff were dispelled by the unit's excellent prospective audit, which is still the only one in the UK to be published on the internet.

However, the surroundings left a little to be desired. The angiography suite is in a new building on one side of the road and has a spanking new ward nearby that's ideal for patients to recuperate in and be closely watched, in case an artery blocks off suddenly (a recognised complication). Alas, the ward has been allocated to Care of the Elderly, which means that following angiography, patients have to go three floors down and into a dark tunnel under the road (known locally as 'the dungeon') and up again to recover on the less than salubrious Ward 20. If their heart stops suddenly, then it's back down to the dungeon and in the lift, with staff furiously pummelling the chest in the hope they can make it back to the angiography suite. The fact that the management have not grasped the idiocy of this situation is symptomatic of their general disinterest in improving the service.

Elsewhere, there are beds in corridors, patients on chairs praying for a bed, and patients in beds who've been waiting for surgery for months. Their plight was bravely championed by Peter Wilde, radiologist and director of cardiothoracic services for the United Bristol Healthcare NHS Trust, who made Tony Blair look like a floundering guppy during the televised debate into the state of the NHS held at St Thomas's in March. He surprised Blair with evidence of big regional differences in funding: 'We have only half the national level of funding for heart surgery, and we have 700 patients on our waiting lists, of which 100 have been waiting for more than a year for open-heart surgery. In the last six months twenty patients have died while waiting for this surgery. We fall not 5% or 3% below the national average; we fall 45% below. We are being committed to waiting-list targets, and yet 70% of our patients are also urgent and need to be operated on immediately.'

The Government has now bunged a few extra million Bristol's way to gloss over the shortcomings in angiography resources, but it has come too late for Wilde, who has resigned his management position in despair. Other consultants talk not just of the lack of central funding, but of the managerial apathy which continually undermines the work of the unit and prevents it from becoming truly innovative.

One Sick Doctor

Hospital doctors too seem to be cracking under the strain. A diagnostic radiologist ('name and address supplied') has written the following letter to the trade magazine *Hospital Doctor*:

> There are a substantial number of patients out there who are unutterably execrable. . . . They are in the main at worst trivially unwell. They need no attention (apart from a good slapping) but insist on being seen. . . . I can only imagine the horror of seeing a waiting room full of these churls and ingrates all bleating louder than sheep, knowing that there is damn-all wrong with them. I have a mental image of revenge – turning to a most loathsome specimen, smiling thinly while declaring, "You've got cancer you bastard – die soon."

Clearly the GMC's insistence that all doctors 'make patients their first concern' has a little way to go.

Lots of Sick Doctors

The Government's National Clinical Assessment Authority (NCAA) was launched this month to help identify (and retrain) 'underachieving doctors'. The NCAA claims that it will give doctors a 'fairer and faster' resolution of complaints against them but there are already 250 doctors on suspension in the UK so it will have its work cut out. Even the GMC accepts that there could be 13,000 drug- or alcohol-dependent doctors out there, waiting to be discovered. The BMA does not trust the Government to help medical addicts and if they were all suspended the NHS would fall to pieces. But the profession's own record in this area is pretty lamentable.

BMA ethics committee member Dr Michael Wilks has been lobbying hard to get the BMA to take addiction seriously, with little progress: 'I have had little success in getting the BMA, the GMC, Royal Colleges and medical defence bodies to invest in a scheme similar to the American "Impaired Physicians' Program". In the USA and Canada, 85–90% of addicted doctors are sober and in work five years after treatment. The Priory would kill for that sort of result. There is also evidence from California that recovering doctors are sued less often than the rest.'

Given that we have so few doctors in the UK, it seems absurd that such a programme isn't up and running in the UK. Perhaps the only hope is for addicted doctors who fall foul of the NCAA to cancel their subscriptions to the BMA and Royal Colleges until they act. If the stocks in the wine cellar start to fall, they'll soon take an interest.

The Bristol Inquiry Finally Reports

20 July 2001

'There are no winners in Bristol. We are all losers.' So said charity director and parent Maria Shortis when the report was finally published last week. But perhaps the biggest losers are the surviving children left permanently brain-damaged by heart surgery. As no unit in the country has kept reliable data on morbidity (i.e. damage short of death), Kennedy was not able to offer any judgement as to whether this was excessive in Bristol compared to an average unit over the eleven years under study. These children have already been forgotten once, by the earlier GMC inquiry, and are offensively recorded in the hospital statistics as 'successes' because they were still alive 30 days post operation.

There are at least 30 such children who need constant care and whose parents face a living hell. Many have a normal life expectancy but because proving clinical negligence is so difficult, they may never receive compensation unless Milburn acts swiftly on Kennedy's suggestion to introduce retrospective no-blame compensation as a gesture of goodwill.

However, ditching negligence litigation before proper mechanisms of accountability are in place in the NHS (which clearly aren't yet), could make it harder to uncover the other Bristol-type disasters that Kennedy believes we can't discount. Were it not for the tenacity of lawyers such as Laurence Vick in the Bristol case, the trust might never have handed over the surgeons' logbooks that helped prove the care was so inadequate.

Another loser in Bristol is the courageous paediatric heart surgeon Ash Pawade, who took over in 1995 when Wisheart and Dhasmana finally threw in the scalpel. Very few, if any, other heart surgeons would have entered such a stressful environment. And yet, immediately, his expertise shone through, despite suffering the same substandard working conditions and split sites as the previous incumbents. While they lost nine out of thirteen babies to the switch operation, he and his colleagues have now performed the operation over 70 times without a single fatality.

The reward for such incredible results should surely be a top merit award, particularly since Wisheart retired with the top A+ grade for services to the profession. Yet despite the promises of health secretaries Dobson and Milburn that these archaic awards would be overhauled to ensure the money goes to those who best serve patients, Pawade has been repeatedly overlooked, along with the equally gifted and progressive adult surgeon Gianni Angelini. Both have done more than anyone to put heart surgery back on the map in Bristol but both, like anaesthetist Steve Bolsin before them, are 'outsiders'. Clearly the club culture is alive and kicking in Bristol and they aren't members.

Outside Bristol, which was rightly praised by Kennedy for publishing its results, the other twelve heart surgery units were also losers for failing to take the opportunity to demonstrate their competence to the public. British Paediatric Cardiac Association president Bob Anderson deserves credit for persuading all the units to at least collect data for the year up to April 2001, which has apparently found that there are no statistically significant poor performers and overall results that are as good as any in the world. However, he wasn't able to release the audit into the public domain because the units hadn't all agreed to it. So we just have to take it on blind trust again. Surely if the information is good enough to reassure us that child heart surgery disasters are no longer occurring, it's good enough for individual units to publish?

Why Doctors Still Make Mistakes

17 December 2001

The Audit Commission's finding that the number of deaths due to drug errors has increased fivefold in the last ten years is no surprise to those who work in the NHS, but the Department of Health's target to reduce these by 40% by 2005 seems a little optimistic. The NHS itself is now one of the leading causes of premature death and disease in this country, with 25,000–40,000 deaths and half-a-million injuries caused each year by preventable errors alone. Labour has decided that promoting a 'no blame' culture will encourage staff to come forward and admit to cockups, enabling swift action to prevent recurrence. But most doctors and nurses still believe that they'll be named and shamed if they own up to anything, as the experience of Andrew Hobart suggests.

Last year Mr Hobart, a newly appointed consultant in accident and emergency medicine at London's Newnham Hospital, turned the wrong knob on an anaesthetic machine and delivered nitrous oxide to the lungs of a three-year-old girl, rather than oxygen. The girl, Najiyah Hussain, died. The anaesthetic machine in question should have been put out of service years ago because such a fatal error is so easy to make under pressure (and has been made before). But obsolete machines get palmed off on casualty departments where no-one would ever need to use nitrous oxide anyway. It's courting disaster, and any doctor could have made that mistake.

An inquiry reached a similar conclusion, recognised Hobart's commitment and compassion and recommended he be allowed to return to work under supervision. So far, so good for the new no-blame culture. However, the *Daily Mirror* has since reported Hobart to the General Medical Council, who are obliged to investigate further, and the Crown Prosecution Service is waiting in the wings to make everyone suffer a lot more. Clearly Hobart's distress cannot compare to that of the Hussains, but if all the doctors who make fatal cockups each year are hung out to dry, the NHS will collapse.

Epileptic Misfit

1 February 2002

The investigation of consultant paediatrician Dr Andrew Holton by the GMC following the alleged misdiagnosis and over-treatment of children with epilepsy at the Leicester Royal Infirmary should provide some indication as to whether the GMC has matured since the Bristol inquiry. In 1998, the GMC nailed Bristol on two surgeons and a manager when the subsequent public inquiry found systemic failures at every level of the NHS. In retrospect, the GMC's impression that this was just a little local difficulty in Bristol looks laughable.

Dr Holton has already run the media gauntlet in our new 'no blame' culture and he may well have made a number of errors, but his working environment was appalling. He was the sole consultant in neuro-developmental paediatrics and, as with the Bristol surgeons, spent many years asking for (and not receiving) extra staffing and resources. His waiting list, especially for EEG (brain-wave) investigation, was ludicrously long and – as with just about every other doctor working in the NHS – there was no-one monitoring his performance and no regular retraining. And although he was working alone, he was certainly not alone in having difficulty with the diagnosis of epilepsy. Across the UK, roughly one in five adults labelled with epilepsy and taking powerful medication for life don't have the disease. And of those who reach the (only) two super-specialist centres in Liverpool and London, the proportion is even higher.

As for treatment of established epilepsy, studies in general practice have shown that many patients are not even seen once a year by their GP, despite picking up repeat prescriptions, and more than 60% could have their treatment improved. So whatever the failings in Leicester, they represent just the tip of a very unpleasant iceberg. As ever in the NHS, the initial barrier to better care is manpower. Recent expert guidelines from the north-west region have recommended that everyone with a possible diagnosis of epilepsy should see a neurologist specialising in the illness within four weeks. The current average waiting time is 28 weeks, and many patients are still being treated by non-specialists and those with inadequate training. At the current level of consultant expansion, the target should be reached by 2019.

A possible solution would be to train specialist GPs to work in community centres to screen all patients with 'fits, faints and funny turns' (over half of whom don't have epilepsy), but this requires both resources and interest from GPs. Epilepsy is extremely stigmatising for patients but viewed by many doctors as dull and boring. None of the twenty specialist registrars currently doing the rounds through the Walton Centre for Neurology and Neurosurgery in Liverpool want to specialise in the disease and most GPs aren't sure who their epileptic patients are and whether they really have epilepsy or not. The disease is just as common as diabetes, but receives a fraction of the media profile and funding because there are no celebrities willing to shout 'I have seizures' from the rooftops.

The situation is particularly desperate in paediatrics, where epilepsy is very hard to diagnose and around a third of children with epilepsy also have learning difficulties such as autism. The need for counselling and support is huge, but rarely are patients followed up into adulthood despite their increased risk of depression and suicide. Whether the GMC focuses on the big picture or on a little local difficulty in Leicester remains to be seen. But as elsewhere in the NHS, changes will probably only occur through litigation. Only about a third of women on anti-epileptic medication are adequately counselled and informed about balancing the risks of the drugs and the risks of seizures to the unborn child. Now, a group of them have hired a lawyer and are suing the NHS for lack of informed consent. Queue the floodgates.

Still Safety Last

15 February 2002

The type of anaesthetic machine that contributed to the tragic death of Najiyah Hussain could inadvertently deliver lethal gas mixture without any oxygen at all. In the early eighties the Canadian Society of Anaesthesiologists made it mandatory for all Canadian machines to be equipped with a mechanism to prevent the delivery of so-called hypoxic gas mixtures. However, a recent survey of 51 NHS hospitals found that 27% did not have 'an anti-hypoxia device'. Most of these were located outside theatre suites, in areas where they would be used infrequently or in emergencies, often by staff not aware of the dangers. Across the NHS, around 3,000 such machines are still in operation.

Replacement of all the machines would clearly be expensive, but would be balanced against the huge personal and financial costs of unnecessary death or brain damage. At the very least, the pure nitrous oxide supply which caused Najiyah's death should be replaced with Entonox, the safe 50:50 mixture of nitrous oxide and oxygen given to labouring women. There are dozens more examples of disasters waiting to happen in the NHS when overstretched staff choose the wrong option. Back in 1987, I nearly killed a patient after I flushed her intravenous line with potassium rather than saline, my defence being that the ampoules looked identical and were stored next to each other. Last year, plastic surgeons at Colchester General Hospital mounted the same defence after mixing up a vial of water with the anaesthetic lignocaine.

This drew an unsympathetic response from Professor Wildsmith of Ninewells Hospital in Dundee: 'To blame the labelling is a diversion of personal responsibility that I find unacceptable because even in a busy plastic-surgery unit, the check takes only a second. ... Don't whinge about the label, read it.' However, with 43% of junior doctors still working above the agreed limit of 56 hours of actual work or 72 hours on-call a week, and most consultants putting in well above their contracted hours, it would be far safer to change the labelling or storage than rely on the 'personal responsibility' of the staff.

Hip Hop

12 April 2002
Would you let someone hammer a great lump of untested metal into the top of your thighbone? It happens every day in the UK. Hip replacements may be one of the success stories of post-war medicine but 10% of them fail to make it to ten years and some pack up much sooner, requiring a much bigger and more painful revision operation. And yet, of the 60-odd different artificial hips used in the NHS and private sector, only a few have good published results over ten years to show that they work. The vast majority are not tested in humans prior to launching and not properly monitored afterwards.

Unsurprisingly, problems aren't picked up until a lot more damage has occurred. Patients given a new hip are reluctant to admit it isn't working and often suffer in silence rather than seek help. Of those that do, 2,000 a year are told their hip prosthesis has failed. The recent recall of the DePuy International prosthesis, because the sterilisation process made it brittle and prone to excessive wear and tear, is one of the few disasters to be picked up. As Professor Chris Bulstrode, an orthopaedic surgeon at Oxford, put it: 'There must be at least twenty hip models currently on the market that are frankly dangerous.'

Back in 1997, I campaigned for a compulsory national register of orthopaedic implants, as in Sweden, to ensure problems were quickly picked up and acted on. Five years down the line, and the rapid-response Department of Health still hasn't decided who should run the registry and even then, reporting won't be mandatory. NICE has at least set targets for hip-prosthesis performance over five and ten years, but unless the audit is properly resourced and mandatory, these will be meaningless.

Most surgeons are too busy cutting waiting lists to monitor their own performance, and in any case, audit should be independently collected to avoid bias. The fact that Labour, for all its bluster about quality, has not even managed to get a compulsory register running to protect patients from unnecessary harm from one of the commonest operations around shows how committed they really are.

Surgeons too are not entirely blameless. As one put it: 'Drug companies are not much different from arms manufacturers. They fly us all out to Florida, pamper us, brainwash us and then get us to use their latest fancy prosthesis.' And once a surgeon's got hooked on a particular gadget, dodgy or not, he tends to stick with it: 'I personally would never use the Ring Hip but I know senior surgeons who still do. It's all they know.'

The absurdity of the current tick-box regulation of prostheses by the Medical Devices Agency (MDA) was exposed by the scandal of the Capital hip, marketed by 3M Healthcare. The MDA can't be bothered to assess products, it just lets manufacturers apply for a stamp of approval from a variety of 'notified bodies' in the EU. Hence, the Capital hip got a meaningless 'CE' mark attesting to its 'non-toxicity' and 'fitness for intended purpose'. It was hammered into 4,700 NHS patients and although the National Audit Office flagged up a possible design fault in 1995, the MDA didn't get round to advising Capital patients to have their hips examined until 1998.

The MDA has introduced a new (voluntary) reporting system for adverse incidents. It's also passing the buck to Europe by asking for legislative changes to ensure better clinical data before a prosthesis is launched, but given that some orthopaedic surgeons have been lobbying for a national register for decades, I wouldn't hold your breath. At present, 70,000 hips are hammered in each year and, isolated enthusiasts aside, we haven't got much of a clue how they're doing until it's too late. When a hip cement called Boneloc was found to have a high failure rate by the Swedish register, it had been used in only fifteen patients. In Britain, it was used on 1,800.

Back in 1993, the *British Medical Journal* warned that the 'fashion trade in joint replacements is costing the health service millions of pounds each year and, even more important, is causing patients unnecessary pain and distress through early failure of unproved implants'. Nearly a decade later, the system of introducing new prostheses is still no more evidence-based than the fashion industry.

So, what should you do if you're waiting for a new hip? The Charnley, Stanmore, Elite and Exeter have good track records. And they wouldn't have stuck any old rubbish in the Queen Mum – she had a Furlong. But the experience of the surgeon is also crucial. A study published in the *Journal of Bone Medicine* in 1996 found that replacements carried out by junior trainees were eleven times more likely to need a revision compared to operations done by consultants. Good luck.

Dr Phil's Notes

There is a national register for orthopaedic implants but it still isn't compulsory. Many NHS orthopods claim that the quality of surgery in some of Labour's new Treatment Centres leaves a lot to be desired, and some have gathered research to prove it. However, their case is weakened by not being able to show that the NHS has got its house in order either. Patients need protecting from sub standard care wherever it occurs.

What, Still No Public Health?

25 April 2002

Hidden away in the Wanless Report is the former bank manager's estimation of the effect of successful reform of the NHS. In 2022, when we may be paying £184 billion a year, the NHS will 'help' to increase life expectancy from 80 to 81.6 years for men and 83.8 to 85.5 years for women. So, a 2% increase over twenty years for all that dosh. This is less to do with the NHS and more to do with the limits of scientific medicine.

In the last century, our life expectancy increased by 30 years but the majority of that was down to improvements in public health. And the biggest challenge facing the UK's health has nothing to do with lack of medicine, but the fact that the rich live ten years longer than the poor. We already have mass involuntary euthanasia – it's called living in the North. A less charitable view is not to blame poverty for the state of our health, but the fact that we've become a population of risk-taking, smoking, alcoholic lard-buckets. Half the NHS budget is deemed to go on illnesses that are (in theory) preventable. Without changing human behaviour, the NHS is doomed.

Alas, the specialty of public health is being decimated by the Labour reforms. District health authorities were abolished in an unseemly rush on April 1, without any clear structure of how to transfer the expertise of public health consultants and non-medical specialists to the new primary care trusts (PCTs), which now control 75% of the budget. Public health resources were already scarce when concentrated in 95 health authorities, but expert teams were built up over years. Now, they're going to be spread across 315 PCTs. In some areas, staff from a single department will now cater for five PCTs. Nearly all their time will be taken up with management and corporate responsibilities, with little time left to develop programmes that might improve public health.

A likely outcome is that PCTs will just cherry-pick the aspects of public health they think they need (e.g. running screening programmes) and overlook the rest. But without the public health expertise to help plan how resources can be more fairly allocated, inequalities will increase. Labour's much-trumpeted NHS Cancer Plan and the National Service Frameworks for other diseases also rely heavily on public health consultants to deliver them.

As one public health consultant put it: 'To say that there must always be change and reform is to forget the fundamental public health questions of what is the evidence for it? And what will be the health impact? Right now, there is considerable evidence that successive reorganisations have been wasteful of time, money and people, and have not delivered service improvement.' As with all political health reforms, Labour's 'biggest shake-up in 50 years' has largely been made up on the hoof, hasn't been piloted and hence there is no evidence to predict whether it will work. However, it will almost certainly have some unpleasant side effects, particularly for public health.

Dr Phil's Notes

The Wanless Report made some good points but, in politics, the medium is the message, and when it was pointed out that Wanless was also a risk manager for Northern Rock, his star waned and opened up the galaxy for Lord Darzi to save the NHS. Darzi's passage was also eased by the waning of chief medical officer Liam Donaldson, one of the architects of the disastrous and unsafe 'career modernisation' of junior doctors.

Depression Special

31 October 2002

Last month, in case you missed it, was the *Rumble in Reno II*, a tense debate at the University of Nevada about the merits (or otherwise) of antidepressants. The original rumble in 2000 claimed that antidepressants don't work nearly as well as the manufacturers claim, but was hampered by the fact that the researchers didn't have access to all the relevant clinical trials. Drug companies have a habit of suppressing 'disappointing' results, but even on the best evidence, it seemed that many antidepressant medications have trouble out-performing sugar pills.

This perception has now been reinforced by the release of the New Drug Application (NDA) data sets from the US Food and Drug Administration (USFDA) for six newer drugs: fluoxetine (Prozac), sertraline, paroxetine (Seroxat), venla-faxine, nefazodone and citalopram. These were obtained under US Freedom of Information legislation and include all the trials the drug companies would rather keep hidden in the filing cabinet. When all the trials are added together, antidepressants offer a very modest two-point reduction in Hamilton Rating Scale for Depression (HAM-D) scores compared to placebos. This difference is statistically, but not clinically, significant, and has been described by researchers as 'a dirty little secret'.

Indeed, in over half of the clinical trials sponsored by drug companies, they failed to find significant differences between the drug and the placebo. In America at least, most experts accept that the average drug/placebo difference in the treatment of depression is very small, and the debate has moved on to how to interpret it and what to do about it. Most doctors still advocate antidepressants as a frontline treatment for severe depression, but the power of direct-to-consumer advertising in the US is such that thousands of Americans take antidepressants for mild depression or just when they're feeling a bit pissed off.

In October 2001, GlaxoSmithKline ran an advertisement in the *New York Times Magazine* for paroxetine (known as Paxil in the United States). A woman is walking on a crowded street, her face strained, in a crowd otherwise blurred. The headline reads: 'Millions suffer from chronic anxiety. Millions could be helped by Paxil.' The fact that this advert occurs so soon after September 11 was surely a coincidence, but prescriptions for antidepressants used to treat both depression and anxiety have increased tenfold in the last decade in both the UK and America. We still lag behind the US when it comes to putting toddlers on antidepressants but it's clear that many patients are still being given a false impression of the power of antidepressants, and worse still, many are told that they are 'easy to come off'.

Earlier this year, the USFDA published a new product warning about severe withdrawal symptoms from paroxetine and the International Federation of Pharmaceutical Manufacturers Associations declared GlaxoSmithKline guilty of misleading the public on US television. And they weren't alone. A few years ago, the Defeat Depression campaign of the Royal Colleges of Psychiatrists and General Practitioners advocated educating patients that discontinuing antidepressant treatment 'will not be a problem'. Even when the issue was recognised, an editorial in the *BMJ* minimised the problems.

Now that the truth is out, most patients will still be wedded to their drugs. They aren't nearly as powerful as you were led to believe but if you try to come off them quickly, the side-effects can be worse than the depression. In the long-term, psychotherapy seems to be a better bet than drugs for mild to moderate depression, with a better long-term cure rate and fewer side effects, but it's extremely hard to get on the NHS. Which is why everyone ends up on drugs.

The Limits of Medicine

24 April 2003

The failure of Labour to turn round the NHS and deliver value for our extra billions is not just because of its flawed model of centralist control using simplistic targets, but it's also down to the over-hyping of medicine. Whatever model of healthcare we have, doubling the amount we spend won't make us twice as healthy, because the treatments don't work as well as the pharmaceutical industry would have us believe. As Richard Smith, editor of the *British Medical Journal*, recently observed: 'Medicine is increasingly about complex and multiple interventions in chronically sick patients with marginal improvements.'

Smith's comments were in response to two studies (*BMJ*, January 11). The first looked at trying to stop elderly patients with dementia who had already fallen, from falling again. 274 patients were assessed by doctors, physiotherapists and occupational therapists, and then one group was randomised to receive intervention on every possible risk factor – including balance, drugs, environmental hazards, feet and footwear, and vision. A huge amount of time and effort went into this study and into the active treatment. And yet the result was no improvement compared with conventional care: three-quarters of patients in both groups fell again, and a fifth died.

A more optimistic study from Aberdeen examined the four-year results of a trial of secondary prevention in over 1,300 patients with coronary heart disease. Patients in the intervention group received multiple tests, treatments and advice. The result after four years was 128 deaths and 125 'coronary events' (e.g. heart attacks) in the control group and 100 deaths and 100 events in the intervention group. A modest success story, but not without considerable effort and organisation usually not available outside the constraints of funded research. Getting that level of care in the NHS is near impossible, and so the real-life benefits of much research are far smaller than claimed.

Further evidence of the huge amount of effort required to eke out small benefits is found in research into cervical screening (*BMJ*, April 25). This is the best model of screening we have and saves 1,300 lives a year. But to prevent one death, we have to screen a thousand women for 35 years. And for each life saved, 150 other women have abnormal results, 80 of whom will be referred on for investigations and possible treatment and one woman will die of cervical cancer despite receiving the best-possible screening. Aside from the organisation and workload involved, even good screening creates large amounts of anxiety and treatment for women who are never going to get cancer. And it only stops half of those who are.

For breast screening, the evidence of benefit is far less. In 2001, a prestigious Cochrane review of all the best available studies led the editor of the *Lancet*, Richard Horton, to conclude: 'At present, there is no reliable evidence, from large randomised controlled trials, to support mammography services.' At best, we have to screen a thousand women over 50 for ten years to save one life, and yet many more suffer the anxiety of abnormal results, invasive breast surgery and chemotherapy for no benefit. The popular perception that a pathologist can always make a clear distinction between cancer and non-cancer has always been false. There is a whole spectrum of cell changes that no-one has a clue as to the significance of, but in a litigious society the 'safe' option is to offer aggressive treatment rather than be held up for missing cancer.

Earlier this year, the *Eye* revealed that in 75% of drug trials, anti depressants are no more effective than placebos. Both work, at least in the short term, but sugar tablets are a lot easier to come off. This provoked a large, predominantly supportive response from *Eye* readers. The respected Critical Psychiatry Network is holding a debate in London on June 3 entitled 'Antidepressants are no better than placebos'.[1] With eminent psychiatrists doubting the very few treatments they have, and Labour favouring coercion and control in their mental-health policy, it's a bad time to be mad.

[1] www.critpsynet.freeuk.com/Press2003.htm

JOHN REID
June 2003–May 2005

The alleged response of Dr John Reid on seeing a panicked Tony Blair on reshuffle morning was: 'Oh fuck, not health.' The response of many NHS staff was: 'Oh fuck, not John Reid.' One self-deluded macho reformer gets replaced with another. But despite the bluster, Reid was far more of a glazier than a window-breaker, largely because he wasn't that interested in the detail and hoped his reward for stepping into the health furnace would be a timely move to defence.

Things looked grim at the outset, with the Commission for Health Improvement announcing a record number of 'zero-star' hospitals and negotiations for GP and consultant contracts in stalemate. But Reid proved very adept at pressing the flesh, and amazed everyone by getting both sets of doctors to sign up to new deals. The secret? Offer them lots of money and let someone else figure out how to pay.

Reid was on a spending spree. He may as well have invited Elton John. He paid private companies over the odds to cherry-pick easy NHS operations and, to cap it all, they got paid top-whack whether they fulfilled their contracts or not. Lots more ludicrously expensive Private Finance Initiative contracts were signed off, and a new system of Payment By Results allowed hospitals to hoover up money. Despite the record investment, the English NHS was heading for record debt, but at least Reid realised it. On his departure, he allegedly advised Tessa Jowell: 'Don't go to health. I've spent all the money.' Reid may have had a PhD, but it wasn't in accounting.

Expenses Update
John Reid used his allowance to pay for slotted spoons, an
ironing board and a glittery loo seat

PRIVATE EYE
Oh Fuck, Not the Working Time Directive

31 July 2003

One of the most pressing issues for new health secretary, Dr
John 'Oh Fuck, Not Health' Reid, is the impending implementation of the European working time directive (EWTD), which
could lead to widespread downgrading of local hospitals and
completely scupper Labour's NHS Plan.

The EWTD requires that by August 2004, junior doctors
should work a maximum of 58 hours a week, with further
restrictions on length of shift, rest periods and sleep while
on-call, falling to 48 hours by 2009. A survey of 211 hospitals
by the Royal College of Physicians has found that 166 'do not
have sufficient numbers of specialist registrars to give
continuous cover of acute medical admissions'. These hospitals
have fewer than ten specialist registrars in medicine, with 44
having fewer than five and, at present, they are completely
unable to cope.

The Royal College of Surgeons has also spotted that a drastic
reduction in hours in the current system will have a dire effect
on training, with many new consultants already unsafe to
independently cover all of the operations in their job
description. But the biggest challenge may be to anaesthetists.
They consume only 3% of hospital resources but contribute to
over two-thirds of trust income. One estimate found that to hit
the targets in the NHS plan and comply with the EWTD, every
graduate from every medical school for the next five years
would need to become an anaesthetist.

The Government has a number of options. It could ignore the legislation and run the risk of mass employment law litigation. It could seek to try to delay the legislation, but is unlikely to succeed. It could 'reconfigure' the NHS, by closing or downgrading lots of smaller district general hospitals and ferrying patients into massive hospitals, which would be politically disastrous and renege on a recent pledge to keep the NHS local. Or it could try and parachute large numbers of junior doctors out of large teaching hospitals and into smaller ones, where most end up as consultants anyway.

The latter seems logical, but many junior doctors deliberately choose to avoid acute general medicine in busy district hospitals because the workload is unremitting, the expectations huge, and support and teaching decidedly variable. Hiding in a teaching hospital, doing research and retreating into a very specialised area of medicine is a far more attractive option.

This is the heart of the battle between the Government and doctors. Labour feels that the NHS employs doctors and should therefore dictate precisely where they work and what that work should involve. Doctors want a degree of professional autonomy, to have the power to challenge politically driven targets and want to be free to choose jobs with humane working conditions and good training. It's a stalemate that even John Reid will have difficulty swearing his way out of.

Anger Management

6 November 2003
A recent BMA survey that found one in three doctors have suffered violent behaviour from patients or relatives of patients in the last year has had some interesting responses. As one casualty registrar put it: 'Is it really only one in three? I've just finished a weekend of nights – physically attacked once,

verbally abused six times, mouthfuls of blood spat at myself and nursing colleagues by one charmer, and the first time our team has been threatened by a gang of fifteen bikers who tried to tear down security screens.'

So, what to do about it? The Government's 'zero tolerance' plan (which involves putting up lots of 'zero tolerance' posters) seems to have failed, so the staff are having to take action. As another casualty doctor put it: 'I've been sworn at, punched, kicked, strangled, threatened with a knife, threatened with being shot (over the phone), had a cigarette stubbed out on my arm, been spat at and attacked with a chair. You have several options while confronted by this:

'1. The "Beirut" approach: I spent two months with Glasgow ambulance paramedics as part of my elective. I was in the back of an ambulance with a paramedic travelling down a 40mph road in Coatbridge when the patient grabbed my collar and started shouting at me. The vehicle screeched to a halt, the back doors flew open and the paramedics threw the patient out of the vehicle onto the road. They then told him if he wanted back in he had to behave himself. Shaken, and meek as a lamb, he climbed back in. Glasgow crews refer to Coatbridge as "Beirut" for this reason.

'2. The "only I get to swear in here" approach: "Shut the fuck up or I'll have you arrested and removed." Make sure you have an open escape route in case the patient decides to attack you.

'3. The "retreat and get the fuzz" approach, returning with them as an escort or outside the curtains. Tell the patient that in view of the threat to your safety you will only treat them with the police present.

'4. The "press charges" approach – I got £100 from a punter on top of his £1,000 fine after he took a chair and chased me round an A&E.

'Once you are happy the patient's life is not in immediate danger, refuse to treat them until they behave. Always make an official report, preferably a police one as well. Document why you were unable to treat the patient properly. And as for aggressive or violent relatives – first sign of trouble and I have them all removed (by the police if necessary).'

Bribing Doctors

30 January 2004

The quality and outcomes framework at the heart of the new GP contract should be a good thing, concentrating on managing chronic diseases better and preventing strokes, heart disease and cancer. But instead of relying on doctors' professionalism to treat patients as best they can, Labour is 'incentivising' them with money. Once you start bribing doctors to behave in a certain way, medicine becomes coercive and the neutrality of professional doctors is undermined. What works for double-glazing doesn't work for diabetes.

As one GP put it: 'Yesterday I went to a meeting about preparing for the new contract. A couple of respected local colleagues gave a presentation on how to earn the most out of it. They explained how they chased up patients via their repeat prescriptions, how their receptionists quizzed people about their smoking habits, and they provided estimates of what they might earn if they hit all their targets. The room was full of intelligent, hard-working, earnest men and women, eager to do their utmost for their patients. But at best they were acting like a bunch of sales reps at a conference, learning how to get out there and flog the product, lapping up all the little tricks of the trade that previously no-one knew of. At worst, they were a bunch of performing seals, expected to jump through hoops and balance beach balls in the hope of someone chucking them a sprat as reward.

'What has my profession come to? No consultant would

stoop this low, to sit and listen to someone tell him his income depended on making his patients sign an "informed dissent" form if they didn't want to take another blood pressure pill. A pox on the General Practitioners' Committee for a contract that reduces us to a bunch of snake-oil salesmen. A pox on all the "yes" voters for agreeing to it. I am thoroughly embarrassed to be part of this.'

Cheap Choice

26 February 2004

The Government's emphasis on increasing patient choice sounds like a vote-winner but will it make the NHS any safer? As GP Dr Nick Summerton warns: 'Choice is not necessarily synonymous with a better-quality service. Patients may choose to have their warfarin treatment monitored in the community, have their skin lesion excised in general practice or have sigmoidoscopy performed in the PCT diagnostic unit. But if the warfarin monitoring service has not signed up to the external quality control scheme, the skin lesion is not submitted for pathological examination or the sigmoidoscope used is rigid rather than flexible, then patients are being short- changed. Sadly these are all real examples. ... An ineffective or unsafe service is not a choice I want to offer to my patients.'

Ex-health minister and now chair of the National Patient Safety Agency (NPSA) Lord Hunt has similar concerns: 'Patients should consider their safety when exercising their right to choice of treatment. Or would they prefer to assume – as they do in the airline industry – that safety is a given and choice can be made on the basis of other factors?' Alas, the NHS is a far more complex and under staffed organisation than the airline industry and safety can never be a given. Each year, 10%

of patients are injured by the NHS, and the equivalent of a jumbo jetload of patients die each week from preventable errors in hospitals alone. Maybe if NHS staff died with our patients, we'd take a bit more care.

Heart surgery is the one example where the NHS is getting its act together in providing meaningful information to patients. It took the Bristol disaster to kick-start it and even then, there is has been huge difficulty in attracting sufficient money for audit. Some centres have managed to translate complex statistics into information that patients can actually use (e.g. Papworth Hospital's newsletters and website http://www.papworth-hospital.org.uk/). Elsewhere it is almost impossible to find accurate, user-friendly information on the safety and quality of NHS services. Without it, the entire patient choice programme could be a huge and very costly stab in the dark.

No Cutting Time

17 June 2004

Would you want to be operated on by a newly qualified consultant surgeon? In a recent poll of the existing crop of senior surgeons, those most in a position to know, an alarming two-thirds said they wouldn't.[1] And further down the tree, the skill levels of junior surgeons have been described as 'very shallow'.[2] The reasoning seems simple enough. In the old days, surgeons worked over 30,000 hours between senior house officer and consultant, gaining a huge amount of experience.

---

[1] Training in the Calman era: What consultants say. *Bull R Coll Surg Eng* 2002; 84(10): 345–7.
[2] An Audit of the Operative Skills of SHOs on BST programmes. *Ann R Coll Surg Eng* 2001; 83(suppl.): S326–7.

Now, it's down to 8,000 hours and will, when the European working time directive comes into full force, fall to 6,000.[3] So new surgeons just don't get the cutting time to pass muster.

Alas, the 'I worked 120 hours a week and it never did me any harm' argument doesn't stand up either. Medicine, and surgery in particular, is littered with the victims of self-imposed workaholism (hence the high percentage of depressed, divorced alcoholics). And as surviving consultant surgeon David Reilly puts it: 'There was no golden age of surgical training. There was certainly more time as a junior doctor; time to mature, or time to rot. And it was apparent that there were some staggeringly bad surgeons appointed under the old system, as well as some highly experienced and motivated ones.'

Also, much of the 120-hour week of old was spent doing meaningless repetitive tasks, propping up the NHS and flying by the seat of your pants, rather than receiving high-quality instruction from your consultant, who often wasn't even in the hospital. However, if we're going to produce competent surgeons in a much shorter time frame, it's clear that a lot of emphasis and resource has to be given to improving the training, and in a ratings-obsessed NHS desperate to cut waiting lists in time for the next election, this just isn't happening.

The largest ever survey of senior house officers in orthopaedic surgery found that a third were not taught at all in theatre or clinic.[4] This is all the more alarming when, by 2010, the NHS is facing a projected 63% increase in knee replacements and a 22% increase in hip replacements. Labour's short-term solution is to farm these operations out to treatment centres, private hospitals and overseas, where there is no obligation to train NHS surgeons. So instead of growing our

---

[3] No Time to Train Surgeons. *British Medical Journal* 2004; 328: 418–19.
[4] Education and Training for SHOs. British Orthopaedic Association 2002.

own talent, we may become utterly dependent on the private sector and abroad.

Trainees often take longer to perform operations, and if a dedicated consultant is supervising them, he or she can't be operating elsewhere. But when the pressure to reduce lists is so great, training just doesn't happen. Consultants are also worried that they carry the can (i.e. position in the published league table) for their trainees' results, and so many are reluctant to let trainees take on anything but the simplest cases.

Even the Royal College of Surgeons has been forced to speak out. As president Sir Peter Morris puts it: 'We have been pressing for dedicated training lists and clinics, regretfully without much success. To deliver training and ensure patient safety with the current staff shortages, existing trainers must be adequately supported with time to teach and train. This will inevitably impact on service throughput.'

Alas, throughput trumps training in Labour's NHS and it's the most junior doctors who suffer. As ex-junior leader Paul Thorpe puts it: 'There is a near total disregard by hospitals of the training needs of SHOs.' The Government can argue that there is no hard evidence that the current crop of new surgeons are any worse than in previous years, but alas in surgery there is very little hard evidence of anything. Despite the fall-out from the Bristol disaster and a clutch of incompetent gynaecologists, not nearly enough resource has gone into improving quality and safety. Instead, Blair is obsessed with treating as many people as possible and offering patients choice to take up spare capacity. But if the choice is between three inexperienced surgeons who don't know what they're doing, is it really worth having?

How to Die

26 July 2004

The verdict of the House of Commons' health committee that 300,000 people each year are denied 'a good death' is old news to the Voluntary Euthanasia Society. The Scottish wing, EXIT, has for some time been running workshops on 'self-deliverance', which include 'the latest how-to methods for dying safely'.

A common misconception for those who wish to end it all is that a single pill will do it quickly and humanely. The human body is generally quite resilient to death. Harold Shipman, whose actions have done incalculable harm to palliative care and the voluntary euthanasia movement, had to use large doses of injected opiates. Similarly, Swiss clinics run by organisations such as Dignitas use large doses of barbiturates.

For those unwilling or unable to fly to Switzerland, EXIT workshops favour a dignified DIY death through slow asphyxiation (cutting off oxygen from the brain). Methods advocated in their July newsletter ('no substitute for attending a workshop') include the use of a ratchet ('available from hardware shops and superstores such as B&Q') to compress the carotid arteries rather than the windpipe ('painful') or just the jugular veins (which leaves your face 'congested and purple').

The ratchet has a 'quick release' tie down which is 'useful for practice runs' but 'make sure you know how to work it properly! Death normally occurs very soon (within minutes) of applying the tie down.' The ratchet method is also 'not for the faint of heart who may be considering, at the back of their mind, a cry for help'.

Another method is to put on a painter's mask and immerse yourself in a very large plastic bag (preferably down to the knees) secured by rubber bands around the neck. The mask stops the bag from obstructing breathing, and so you achieve a gentler unconsciousness. You can also use a pair of tights and a wooden spoon to deliver yourself. You turn the spoon to tighten the neck ligature of the tights: 'Bending forward increases the diameter of the neck and thus the constrictive effect of the tights ... the method can be achieved relatively unobtrusively – some small convulsions are likely between passing out and death, but it might pass easily unnoticed.'

That there is a need for these workshops at all is a sad reflection on our treatment of the irreversibly and terminally sick. Very few people wish to be seen shitting and pissing the bed in front of the family when their mind's gone to putty, and yet thousands suffer degrading and prolonged deaths each year. And those who engage in mercy killings, such as 100-year-old Bernard Heginbotham, still get hauled through the courts.

For all Labour's guff about extending patient choice, the one area where it truly matters – when, where and how you die – is still a huge political taboo that is pushed to the back of the queue. 55% of deaths still occur in hospital, when most people express the wish to be at home, and palliative care provision is alarmingly unequal. For example, North Yorkshire gets 20,500 hours of Marie Curie nursing a year but West Yorkshire – four times the size – gets only 11,000. And after Shipman, we'll need to double the non-existent nurses to go through all the drug-safety checks. No wonder people are reaching for the ratchet.

Returning to Practice

24 August 2004

My recent return to general practice seems an apt time to reflect on the state of the National Health Service. It isn't national, it's not a coherent service and it's got very little to do with health. Patients still come in with ear wax and self-limiting illness, and about half of them are overweight. Some of those that need referral onwards are sent to privately owned treatment centres, often without their GP's knowledge. Even though it's our duty to make sure patients get a good service, we're given no information as to the safety and quality of the treatment. But at least it's quicker.

Like the rest of the NHS, general practice itself is being carved up into hundreds of individual tasks which can then be individually coded and costed as a prelude to privatisation. In theory, GPs can then choose whether they wish to do a task for the price offered (e.g. monitor patients on blood-thinning drugs) but in order to claim the fee, they have to stick to strict protocols and keep meticulous, repetitive records. If they choose to opt out, their local PCT is obliged to open the market to other providers, often private, who think they can do the job at that price. The results are predictable; companies will cherry-pick easy cases but complicated ones will get bounced back to the GP.

GPs could refuse, but in practice it's hard to turn down a distressed and confused elderly patient with multiple illnesses and tablets who is in danger of having a major bleed if she gets the dose of warfarin wrong. In a sense, GPs have for decades been their own worst enemies by providing an extensive, holistic but largely unmonitored service much more cheaply than any private company could do. And although a majority of GPs signed up to their new contract, many did so for the chance of opting out of 24-hour responsibility for their patients, rather than a desire to anally document and claim for each of the vast range of tasks they've been doing anyway since the inception of the NHS.

Labour's NHS has become entirely preoccupied with treating diseases, modifying risks and counting all there is to count, rather than focusing on the outcomes that matter. Many patients benefit from simply having someone who listens and accepts them as they are. Most GPs hate being judgemental and forcing medicalisation on people who don't want it, because study after study shows it doesn't work (for example, only a third of patients on long-term medication take it properly). Patients want more face-to-face time with GPs, but they're getting less, and consultations are now interrupted with 'We'd better just pop you on the scales' and 'Do you mind if I just check your blood pressure?' It then takes another five minutes putting all these numbers into the appropriate computer template to claim the fee for measuring them.

GPs now see fewer patients than they used to and fill the time with administrative and management tasks to justify their value to the Government. But the true value of what they do has always been rooted in empathy and support and all the other fluffy things that we can't easily measure. All the extra investment in the NHS is giving us a lot more numbers to count and regale us with come election time, but I doubt the patients are getting much healthier and the GPs are grumpy as hell at being forced to administer a style of doctoring they don't believe will work. Apart from that, it's great to be back.

PATRICIA HEWITT
May 2005–June 2007

Poor Patsy. Lumbered with the bill for John Reid's spending spree, she had to somehow explain how a health service with record investment could end up in record debt. She came up with some memorable soundbites. 'The NHS has never had it so good' went down so well at the Royal College of Nursing that she was booed and slow hand-clapped by those worried about job cuts. But my favourite quote was: 'A penny wasted in the NHS is a penny stolen from a patient.' This from a government that spent billions on an IT system that hasn't delivered, commercial building contracts that were too secret to scrutinise, sweeteners to open the doors of the NHS to private competition, and management consultants to disguise what was happening from the Labour faithful. Then add in the costs of administrating a continuous and contradictory reform programme. (Establish primary care trusts, then close them down again. Abolish GP fundholding, then build it up again. Build lots of new hospitals, then take as much work as possible away from them.) You have to at least admire her brass neck.

Hewitt tried her best to pin the blame on greedy GPs, but it was the Department of Health who had agreed the deal with the consent of Blair and Brown, despite warnings from the BMA negotiators that most GPs would easily hit the targets set for them. Unlike Reid, Hewitt was good with accounts and managed to get the NHS back into the black, causing a lot of resentment and anger on the way. She also had to cop it for the junior doctor job-application fiasco, and paid for it with her own job. No-one loves an accountant, especially one with an accountant's communication skills.

PRIVATE EYE
Don't Believe What You Read

25 August 2005

Should we trust what we read in esteemed medical journals? And are they any good at identifying medical fraud? The answers to both may be 'no', if you believe a recent survey of journal editors carried out by the *BMJ* for the Committee on Publication Ethics. Most journals do not have policies for dealing with misconduct, nor do they have complaints procedures for handling allegations, despite a series of scandalous publications (such as the cloning breakthroughs claimed by Korean scientists).

As Dr Fiona Godlee, editor of the *BMJ*, put it: 'Biomedical journals often have few resources available to them and little in the way of back-up, added to which for many journal editors, the role is part-time. This often makes it very hard for them to pursue matters further. Nevertheless, complaints procedures and guidance for authors should be standard minimum requirements for journals.'

At present, it seems we can't spot the cheats and liars who harm patients and waste money to further their own careers. As Richard Smith, former editor of the *BMJ*, once put it: 'Half of what appears in medical journals is excessive, bent or crummy.' The trouble is, it's hard to spot which half before publication. Smith also believes that medical journals are just an extension of the pharmaceutical industry.[1] Many now carry drug adverts but he does not see this as the main problem. Although it's a clear signal of a journal's financial dependence on the industry, ads are so upfront and conspicuous that they're easy to disregard. Much harder to spot is the bias of industry-sponsored randomised controlled trials: 'Readers see

---

[1] www.plosmedicine.org May 2005; Volume 2 Issue 5.

randomised controlled trials as one of the highest forms of evidence. A large trial published in a major journal has the journal's stamp of approval and may well receive global media coverage. . . . A company will sometimes spend upwards of a million dollars on reprints of the trial.'

Amazingly (or not), studies funded by a company are four times more likely to have results favourable to the company than studies funded from other sources. So how do drug companies manage to get the results they want? The tactics, according to Smith, are numerous. You can conduct a trial of your drug against a treatment known to be inferior. Or trial your drugs against too low a dose of a competitor drug. Or use too high a dose (making the competitor seem toxic). You can use multiple endpoints and just publish the one that's favourable. Or do multi-centre trials ands just publish the favourable centres, or even just publish a subgroup that seems to work.

The bottom line, however, is to construct the trial well enough to get into peer-reviewed journals, which only drug companies have the resources to do. Between two-thirds and three-quarters of the trials published in the major journals are funded by the industry. But if the industry doesn't fund this research, who will? Higher taxes for more publicly funded research. Now there's a vote-winner.

Non-Sexy Illnesses No. 456 – Blackouts

8 September 2005
Around 30% of patients diagnosed with epilepsy actually suffer from a disturbed heart rhythm (arrhythmia), which leads to a temporary loss of consciousness resembling a seizure. Some patients suffer many such attacks of 'reflex syncope' in a short space of time, which is very debilitating and distressing, and yet

many go for years without the correct diagnosis or treatment. The lucky few who are diagnosed can be very effectively treated with a pacemaker.

A consultant cardiologist and *Eye* reader describes one such patient who was misdiagnosed with temporal lobe epilepsy for 27 years. She suffered severe bouts of depression and avoided socialising for fear of having an attack. She had to reduce her working week to eighteen hours, was unable to swim alone and received very little help from the NHS.

'Despite her appalling suffering she experienced off-hand treatment at the hands of unmotivated clinicians hiding within a dysfunctional and unresponsive system. Her local neurologist laughed at her, the cardiologist wouldn't deign to see her, and the local commissioner wouldn't agree to her having a pacemaker in London.

'In desperation, she came to me in my private rooms (her GP having refused to refer her to my NHS clinic). I did not charge her. I asked her husband to leave the room, told her to feign a blackout, admitted her to my NHS hospital and put in a pacemaker that afternoon. Since that time she has got a completely new life, with work, friends, exercise and new confidence.'

The consultant, who wishes to remain anonymous, believes the outlook for patients with unsexy illnesses that aren't targeted or given extra resources remains poor. 450 people per million receive pacemakers in the UK for the treatment of slow heart rhythms, compared to an average of 900 in Western Europe. Similarly, only 45 UK patients per million receive implantable cardioverter defibrillators to protect them from sudden cardiac arrest compared to 85 in Western Europe. And France, Germany and Italy also have five times as many electrophysiologists (heart-rate specialists) as the UK.

The top-down, centralist NHS will never be able to treat patients according to clinical need while resources are so unevenly distributed and patients have very little clout in seeking out the treatment they need. Those suffering from recurrent blackouts would be well advised to visit the Syncope Trust and Reflex Anoxic Seizures website (www.stars.org.uk).

Unsexy Illnesses No. 898 – Cystic Fibrosis

17 November 2005

In April 2001, public health minister Yvette Cooper announced a national neonatal screening programme for cystic fibrosis (CF), the UK's most common, life-threatening inherited disease. So why hasn't it happened yet? Biochemical screening for CF has been available in the UK since 1980, and newborns served by laboratories in East Anglia, Trent, Northampton and Leeds have been screened for some years, as have those in Northern Ireland, Wales and Scotland. An England-wide service was due to be rolled out last year, led by the UK Newborn Screening Programme Centre, but four and a half years after Cooper's promise, it still hasn't arrived.

Screening has become more important as treatments for CF have improved. In CF, the lungs and pancreas can get clogged with thick sticky mucous and in the 1930s, when the disease was first recognised, 70% of babies died within a year. Now, thanks to the development of specialist paediatric and adult CF centres, and the combination of early diagnosis and swift treatment, patients can live into their forties.

In the absence of screening, many patients are diagnosed late, if at all. One in 25 of us carry the faulty CF gene, and statistically, there are 2.3 million carriers of the faulty gene and 7,500 people with CF in the UK. However, only 6,000 are currently treated in specialist centres. The remaining 1,500 are either as yet undiagnosed or being treated by non-specialists, who see only a few cases a year and lack the expertise and resources to do it properly. There has been published evidence for seven years that specialist centres get better results,[1] because they treat very aggressively to maintain maximum weight and lung function. However, they cannot reverse the damage done by inadequate treatment or late diagnosis. A screening programme that channelled all affected babies into specialist care would help resolve this.

Alas, CF is not a high-priority illness, and research by the CF Trust a year ago found that a third of patients have trouble getting the best drugs and treatments even at specialist centres. Not one of the 38 centres provided 'recommended levels of care', and only nine were able to employ even half the staff they needed. The overall shortfall in funding for CF care was estimated at 50%. At present, indebted PCTs can simply refuse to pay for proper CF care for their patients, which may explain the delay in screening. What's the point in identifying more babies with CF if you aren't going to commit the resources to providing the best treatment?

Meanwhile, £17.5 billion of NHS funding is being put aside for the private sector for absurdly expensive and inflexible PFI contracts and £6.2 billion has been committed to an NHS IT superhighway that has thus far delivered very little. Indeed, according to its boss Richard '£250,000 a year' Granger, it is 'in grave danger of being derailed'. Here's a thought. Give the money back to patients.

Swallow That

9 February 2006

The revelation, courtesy of the Commission for Social Care Inspection, that the elderly are given the wrong drugs in half of all care homes could be construed as progress; when left to

---

[1] Clinical outcome in relation to care in centres specialising in cystic fibrosis. *British Medical Journal* 1998; 316: 1771–5 (13 June).

their own devices only a third of patients take their tablets properly. This long-standing problem has been compounded of late by the absurd number of pills elderly patients have to pop so GPs can hit the Government's targets and send their children to public school.

Targets do at least concentrate the mind but as Peter Winocour, a consultant NHS diabetologist puts it: 'targets are often impractical and involve taking too many drugs . . . 10% of type 2 diabetics could require two or three hypoglycaemic agents (ultimately including insulin), at least three antihypertensive agents, two hypolipidaemic agents, and aspirin. A high proportion will also require treatment for coexistent cardiovascular disease and coincidental unrelated chronic disease. It is difficult to see how we can realistically expect patients to comply for long with such a draconian regimen requiring so many separate drugs.'[1]

To illustrate the point, a GP has written to the *Eye* about an elderly woman who was expected to take twenty tablets of sixteen different drugs spaced out over four different time intervals: 'One of the drugs was warfarin, to reduce the risk of stroke, which interacted with a lot of the other drugs and required regular blood tests (INRs) to get the correct dose. However, the INR was wildly variable and we couldn't get the dose of warfarin right. It later transpired that instead of adhering to her absurdly complicated drug regime, she'd tipped all sixteen bottles of tablets into a basket and swallowed twenty at random each day, figuring out it would all even up in the end.'

Given the increasing pill burden of the elderly (as we try to keep them well enough to travel to Switzerland to end their lives), care home staff need more than training to get the tablets

---

[1] Winocour P. Effective diabetes care: a need for realistic targets. *BMJ* 2002; 324: 1577–80.

right, they need someone with the time to do nothing else all day but dish them out.

Moneybags GPs?

19 April 2006

As a GP, I earn £40 an hour. To take home £250,000 a year, as the BBC is suggesting, I'd need to clock up 120 hours a week. I used to do this as a junior doctor, but I was knackered and dangerous. Any GP still putting in those sorts of hours is welcome to the money, although he (and it probably is a he) is also likely to be knackered and dangerous.

This furore over GPs' pay is a convenient smokescreen for Labour's failure to radically improve the NHS. The current debts are not because the reforms are 'biting', but rather because they haven't happened. Getting access to, or time with, the GP you choose is harder than it ever was. And consultations are now driven by targets, not patients.

When I qualified in 1990, I had ten-minute appointments. Today, I still have ten-minute appointments. The patients are equally complicated but more likely to demand and complain (unsurprisingly, given the money going into the NHS). Doctors need time to diagnose and treat safely, patients need it to express themselves, but neither get it. So where's the reform?

As Professor Aidan Halligan, the director of clinical governance for the NHS in England and former deputy chief medical officer put it: 'We have learnt that throwing money at the problem only allows us to do more of what we have always done. Any suggestion of real reform has been a deceit.

'Targets have become an end rather than a means and, together with blinkered performance management, have distorted healthcare priorities. . . . At a moment of unprecedented need, healthcare is suffering a leadership void which has caused it to lose its way.'

Centrally imposed market reforms can never work, not least because the vast majority of the NHS workforce believe health is a right, rather than a commodity. Although GPs, and the drug industry, are earning more for lumbering patients with twenty tablets a day that they can't possibly remember to take, the vast majority of NHS funding still goes into hospitals. The Tories allowed some GPs to develop better community services (and higher wages) through fundholding, but it was an iniquitous system that penalised patients of non-fundholders. However the ethos of providing cheaper, better care for patients outside hospitals was correct.

Alas Labour, having preached the evils of fundholding in opposition, could not draw on its strengths and extend it to all. So it was abolished. Now, nine years later, fundholding has been resurrected as practice-based commissioning, but now all the new money has been gobbled up (largely by hospitals) and the NHS is rife with debt, panic and job insecurity. In such a climate, it can only fail.

For nine years, Blair's main focus has been on waiting times for hospital treatment, which were eighteen months when he took over and which he hopes will be eighteen weeks when he leaves. This would be an undoubted improvement, at huge cost, but given that over 90% of healthcare has nothing to do with hospitals, it hardly represents system reform. Instead, we've had nine years of lurching between contradictory initiatives and – surprise, surprise – we've hardly moved at all. Time to blame those greedy GPs.

Placebos For All

1 June 2006

The exhortation of thirteen senior consultants that the NHS should desist from funding unproven alternative therapies (*The Times*, May 23) was a touch biased, given that many conventional treatments are also of dubious benefit. According to *Clinical Evidence* (www.clinicalevidence.com), only 15% of the thousands of treatments they have reviewed have been proven to be beneficial. A further 23% are likely to be beneficial, 7% are a trade-off between benefits and harms, 5% are unlikely to be beneficial, 4% are likely to be ineffective or harmful and a whopping 46% are of 'unknown effectiveness'. Clearly, much more research needs to be funded before the NHS can claim to be evidence-based.

Surgery is impossible to subject to the gold standard 'double-blind randomised controlled trial' since any surgeon worth his salt knows if he is performing a proper or sham operation. But the placebo effect is just as evident in surgery as it is in homeopathy. Patients with osteoarthritis who are tricked into thinking their knee joint has been washed out and the bits removed have as much pain reduction and improved movement as those who've had proper arthroscopy.[1] For decades, orthopaedic surgeons have earned a fortune just by blowing air into joints.

There is no doubt that the vast majority of complementary therapies also operate on the placebo effect. In the few trials where acupuncture or homeopathy have been shown to work, it doesn't much matter what remedy you give or where you stick the needles. What matters is the strength of the relationship between therapist and client, and the belief, expectation and suggestion that goes with it. One reason it costs drug companies nearly a billion dollars to get a new drug to market is the great difficulty many of them have in out-performing a placebo.

Placebos produce noticeable improvements across a whole range of symptoms and illnesses, such as pain, tiredness,

[1] Moseley et al. *New England Journal of Medicine* 2002; 347: 81–8.

nausea, high blood pressure, angina, asthma, hay fever, head-aches, PMT, depression, anxiety, peptic ulcers, high cholesterol, insomnia, hot flushes and social problems. They can reduce the frequency of epileptic seizures, have nasty side-effects and reverse the effects of powerful drugs. Placebos even work if you tell patients that's what they're taking. In one study,[2] fifteen psychiatric patients suffering from neurotic symptoms were told: 'We feel that a so-called sugar pill may help you. Do you know what a sugar pill is? A sugar pill is a pill with no medicine in it at all. I think this pill will help you as it has helped so many others. Are you willing to try this pill?' Fourteen said yes and thirteen improved during the week, some a great deal, including one previously suicidal patient.

All medicine is in large part placebo, yet some doctors are jealous of the complementary therapists' freedom to 'big up' their placebo effect by talking unscientific bollocks. But far from wasting money, complementary therapy does in many cases save it by avoiding the prescription of more expensive, and potentially harmful drugs. In a free-at-the-front-door health service, patients flood in with all manner of bizarre symptoms and emotional hang-ups that science has yet to find an answer for. Without complementary therapy, patients end up on Prozac or painkillers just to get them out of the door.

The only other alternative is counselling, which has some evidence base but it's used by GPs to pass the buck. As Dr Phil Peverley puts it: 'Our referral letters essentially say the same thing: "Dear counsellor, I don't want to talk to this patient any more. You do it." . . . Our counsellor was a proper nurse until three months ago, but she is now trained to listen to any old shite without laughing.'[3]

---

[2] Park L, Covi L. Non blind Placebo Trial. *Archives of General Psychiatry* 1965; 12: 336–45.

[3] Peverley. *Pulse Magazine* 1 June 2006.

Alas, I can't practise complementary therapy without laughing ('you've got too much jitsu in your tsubo . . .') but I know plenty of people who can. The NHS would implode without them.

Regulating Doctors

26 July 2006

What's the best way to regulate doctors? No-one seems to know, least of all the chief medical officer Liam Donaldson. His post-Shipman review (*Good Doctors, Safer Patients*), is full of the same rhetoric as its post-Bristol predecessor (*Supporting Doctors, Protecting Patients*), and its scatter-gun approach of 44 recommendations could just add a hugely expensive 'scrutiny bureaucracy' without making doctors better or patients safer.

Donaldson's most contentious suggestion is for the burden of proof in actions against doctors to be lowered from criminal ('beyond reasonable doubt') to civil ('on the balance of probability'). This may pick up doctors who are dangerous for patients but not too dangerous for the GMC, but it may also result in mass suspensions and a surge in defensive medicine where doctors over-investigate and refer rather than take the buck themselves. This would be extremely expensive and counter to the Government's aim of getting GPs to accept more responsibility and minimise hospital care.

Donaldson also wants doctors to be re-licensed every five years, rather than just once on qualification and never again thereafter. This sounds reasonable, and indeed I underwent a form of re-licensing last year when I returned to general practice after a career break. It consisted of a knowledge-based multiple choice questionnaire (MCQ), two hours of video consultations and a structured trainer's report. I passed, but then again the tests are hard to fail. The MCQ is positively marked, so a monkey with a pencil would get 50% by chance alone. The video does not have to be continuous, so you can exclude any consultation where you've cocked up badly. And trainers have a habit of passing their trainees, lest it reflect badly on their teaching.

What matters is not whether doctors can jump through the artificial hoops of exams (most can, which is how we became doctors in the first place) but whether the consequences of our everyday actions lead to avoidable harm for patients. The most useful scrutiny I have had is the analysis of my actions by other doctors, particularly the cockups and near misses. For example, I recently diagnosed a patient's chest pain as non-cardiac, based on the history. Four months later, he had a heart attack.

Like any other doctor, I want to know if I got it wrong and, if so, what I should do to get it right next time. Most GP practices and hospitals have regular significant-event audit meetings; some are rigorous and at times brutal, but others tend to be too uncritical for fear of upsetting colleagues. What's needed are doctors in every region, who are independent of the medical establishment, to analyse potential errors in a fair and balanced way. Both doctors and patients would then get quick, impartial feedback. And those doctors who repeatedly err would be picked up earlier.

I first argued for an independent medical inspectorate focusing on errors in 1999.[1] Sir Liam's answer is to introduce local, medically qualified 'GMC affiliates', paired with a public buddy. But without true independence, it seems no more likely to succeed than the 'Assessment and Support Centres' he proposed seven years ago.

Politicians don't trust doctors to regulate themselves in secret, but neither do doctors trust politicians or the GMC to do it fairly and competently. The key question is 'Who picks up doctors' mistakes?' If it's done independently, swiftly and fairly,

[1] See Pickering W. in *Regulating Doctors*. ISBN 1–903–386–0

we'll all benefit. If it becomes a political process, where good doctors are defined as those who do what Labour wants them to, it'll be a disaster.

There's Only Four NHSs

26 July 2006

During the last election, Tony Blair took the piss out of the Welsh health service for its long waiting times compared to England. Given that Wales is theoretically served by the same National Health Service that Blair had promised to turn around it seemed a brave call, and one that caused huge embarrassment to Welsh Labour MPs. But the Welsh Assembly has chosen to take their NHS in a different direction from Blair's relentless focus on competition and privatisation in England. In Wales, the emphasis is on tackling the causes of ill health, rather than trying to micromanage the NHS. So who'll have the last laugh?

Instead of spending hundreds of millions of pounds abolishing community health councils, setting up a Commission for Public and Patient Involvement in Health and closing it down again, Wales simply kept the CHCs. It has invested in free breakfasts for primary school children and free prescriptions for all. Devolved parliament in Scotland has funded free personal care for the elderly, whereas in England thousands of elderly patients are denied nursing care on the NHS because their medical needs are artificially reclassified as 'social' and they have to sell their homes to pay for care.

The Scottish Parliament also managed to reconfigure its health services with broad support from the public and health service staff, in marked contrast to the divisive battles over privatisation that the English NHS is enduring. In Wales and Scotland, the ethos is more to trust professionals to do their jobs out of a sense of vocation, rather than rely on market forces and excessive regulation to do it for them. PCTs, payment by results, star ratings, compulsory choice and practice-based commissioning do not even exist in Wales or Scotland. And the hugely bureaucratic raft of proposals that Sir Liam Donaldson introduced to revalidate doctors only applies to England.

The downside for Wales and Scotland is that their left-wing, increasingly nationalist approach has ducked the politically combustible issue of hospital closures. In Wales, the mindset is that each area should offer uniform services, which is neither efficient nor cost-effective. In Northern Ireland hospital activity is 26% lower than England per bed. Scotland is using the private sector to get waiting lists down, though much less so than England and only when there is a real need (as opposed to the English stance of competition for the hell of it).

Scotland's reform programme seems to be the most co-ordinated, with its focus on networks and partnerships. In Wales, first minister Rhodri Morgan is aiming for 'clear red water' between Cardiff and London and the Lib Dems are too supine to object. In England, the volume and haste of new initiatives, some of which directly contradict others, has meant that not even senior managers are clear about what they're supposed to be aiming for.

What is clear is that there is no UK focus in health policy, and there are huge disparities in entitlement and treatment across four countries. This is completely contrary to the notions of equity and treatment according to need, and it'll be some years before we discover who got it right. The three smaller countries at least have the advantage of watching the English NHS crash and burn, and then cherry-picking the good bits. In the meantime, go to England for quick operations, Wales for free prescriptions, Scotland for long-term care and Northern Ireland if you don't like change.

Indiscreet Doctors

7 September 2006

Would you let someone who claims to be a doctor examine you, without any pretence of privacy, on a crowded high street? And let it be filmed? Fortunately for the makers of *Street Doctors* (*The One Show*, BBC1, September 4–8), there are plenty of people who will. But can you give informed consent to a televised medical ambush?

My worst experience of this was presenting *As it Happens* for Channel 4, live from City Hospital in 1997. The producer was desperate to film cardiac resuscitation, and reckoned he could get consent too: 'We'll put a two-minute delay on the filming and if the resuscitation's successful, we'll get the patient to sign the release form when he comes round.' Mercifully, it never happened.

A year later, BBC1 released *The Human Body*, fronted by Robert Winston, which managed to get a dying man to consent to filming his death, a BBC researcher to consent to thermal imaging of his erect penis and pregnant women awaiting terminations to consent to intra-uterine filming of foetal development.

In 2002, BBC3 pushed the boundaries further with *Sex, Warts and All*, a much praised series on sexual health which somehow got patients to admit to having sexually transmitted infections and to show their genitals (warts and all) to the camera. As adviser Dr Rak Nandwani put it, 'It's had a great impact in reducing the stigma of sexual health clinics, and has encouraged people to attend.'

Destigmatisation is the standard defence of all medical confession programmes, but rarely is much thought given to the consequences of such public exposure. On *Street Doctors*, a man at a fruit and veg market was found to have a blood pressure of 188/109, which is certainly worth knowing about.

But do you want to share it with your employer or insurer?

In 2004, I was asked to comment on the health of the 'volunteers' for BBC1's *Fat Nation*, filmed live from a street in Birmingham. The producer had assembled a spreadsheet of coronary risk factors (blood pressure, cholesterol, smoking and diabetic status) that the inhabitants had apparently consented to having read out on BBC1 when signing their release forms. The results were so shocking, with half the street likely to suffer a heart attack or worse in the next decade, that the item was dropped because it didn't fit in with the happy clappy 'let's get fit together' ethos.

Back on *Street Doctor*, fruit and veg man is told his blood pressure is '8 out of 10' on a scale of badness, whatever that means. Another woman is told she might have rheumatoid arthritis as she leans on her burger bar and a boy is undressed to find he has 'molluscum contagiosum' under his arm: 'Nothing to worry about,' claims Doctor Barbara, though whether he'll see it that way in the playground the morning after transmission is debatable.

Inevitably, a man takes his trousers off and squats on a bag of shallots to be examined, but even more undignified was a man lying on a mat with his head resting on the kerb. Most of what gets dished out is reassurance, but medicine has a habit of dishing out nasty surprises and examining a pregnant woman in the middle of Bury market would be disastrous if the foetal heartbeat was absent.

The GMC and BMA agree on very few things, but patient confidentiality is one of them. Bizarrely, one of the street doctors is George Rae, who in July came second in a vote to become chairman of the BMA and is now wandering around Manchester exhorting patients to strip off in public and 'worry yourself not'. Come back Frankie Howerd.

Doctors and the Drug Industry

6 October 2006

Does the drug industry still have too much influence over doctors? I was asked to support this motion, with Labour MP Howard Stoate, at the Oxford Union last month. The debate was paid for by the industry and attended by its employees, so unsurprisingly we lost. But I left £500 richer (plus expenses, meal and overnight accommodation).

Opposing us were two GPs, Peter Fellows and George 'street doctor' Rae, current and former Chairmen of the BMA prescribing sub-committee. Their (paraphrased) argument is that medicine is now so closely scrutinised and regulated, with prescribing largely dictated by evidence-based formularies, that it's far harder for doctors to wander off-message and prescribe bucket-loads of an unproven drug because they like the breasts of a cheerleader rep. Besides, doctors are professionals who are trained to absorb any amount of excessive hospitality without it clouding our professional judgement.

Indeed, the days of excessive hospitality are supposed to be over, thanks to the new Association of the British Pharmaceutical Industry (ABPI) code that came into effect on January 1, 2006. Freebies given to doctors, otherwise known as 'promotional aids', should cost no more than £6 (excluding VAT). This should be the street value, so a company can't bulk buy 20,000 rubber nun suits with 'Pfizer' tattooed above the buttocks if I can't buy the same item in my local corner shop for £6 or less.

Also, the gift has to be relevant to professional practice. Branded thermos flasks, travel rugs, teapots, dentures, barometers etc. are out. And the gift has to be matched to the recipient. For example, a rep can't give a receptionist a tongue depressor (even if she's really earned one). Travel expenses can't be paid for local meetings and all flights are economy only (unless you're a speaker). You can't take your wife, lover or children unless there's a good professional reason for it. There are dozens more rules ranging from the size of the lettering on 'laminated leave pieces' to the format of the inane adverts placed in medical journals. And unlike medical self-regulation, where very few people shop a colleague, competitors are lining up to report you if you stray from the code.

The downside is that membership of the ABPI isn't compulsory, and given that most doctors haven't got a clue who's in and who's out, suspension seems only to cause a little internal embarrassment. On February 10, 2006, Abbott Laboratories were suspended from the ABPI for 'a minimum of six months' after being rumbled taking doctors on various corporate jollies (one to Wimbledon and two to a greyhound racing stadium). However, it was the escort of a doctor to an evening presentation with two leading-edge female presenters (i.e. a lap-dancing bar) that raised the most eyebrows.

Abbott don't seem to have suffered commercially for their slapped wrist and indeed they were reinstated to the ABPI on July 1, less than five months into their minimum six-month suspension. Overall, the drug industry in the UK spends £1.65 billion marketing its drugs, whereas the Department of Health spends just £4.5 million a year providing independent prescribing information to doctors (or at least it did until it axed its subscription to the excellent *Drugs and Therapeutics Bulletin*). Drug companies pay for or subsidise just about every educational meeting doctors attend. They wouldn't do it without some return.

One solution would be for doctors to pay for their own education, or at least for the industry to pool its educational grants so no individual company has undue influence over training. But all this is pointless if we can't trust the 'evidence' on which our training is based. The drug industry is certainly clearing up its front-of house operations, but companies still control the research and information flow about their own products, and they use medical journals as an extension of their marketing arm. If all companies were obliged to pool their clinical-research funding, so that all large-scale trials could be performed and published independently of the manufacturer, we'd all be a lot safer.

Statins for All?

20 October 2006

Should you try to get your cholesterol as low as possible? What you eat has very little bearing on your blood level of 'bad cholesterol' (LDL), so the only way to reduce it is to take statins. This would certainly please the pharmaceutical industry, which already makes more than £20 billion a year on this class of drug, but is anyone swallowing it?

Statins are the biggest-selling drugs ever, and by inhibiting an enzyme involved in the liver synthesis of cholesterol, they reduce the level of circulating cholesterol in the bloodstream. If you already have heart disease, or lots of risk factors for it (diabetes, high blood pressure, smoking), there is good evidence that statins reduce your risk of 'future cardiac events'. It's assumed they do this by stopping the build-up of rancid LDL in the walls of your arteries but some studies show they cut the risk of heart disease independently of their effect on cholesterol. However they work, they reduce the risk of nasty things happening to your heart. The key questions are which patients should take a statin and how much?

In the UK, GPs are 'incentivised' (i.e. bribed) by the Government to get the total cholesterol of patients with heart disease and stroke (or at 30% risk of having either in the next decade), down to 5 mmol/l or less. This doesn't make much sense, since you need to know how much of it is good (HDL) or bad (LDL) but these tests are more expensive so we lump it all together. As a result, two and a half million UK patients are already on statins, at an average annual cost of over £150 each. GPs get their payments if they get 60% of their patients to target. Some patients, particularly those at much higher risk with very high cholesterol levels, are harder to treat but provided a GP has ticked off the easy 60%, there's no financial incentive to treat the patients who need it most.

Recently, the Joint British Societies have recommended a target total cholesterol of 4 mmol/l and an LDL of less than 2 mmol/l in high-risk groups. The US National Cholesterol Program recommends an even tougher target of 1.81 mmol/l. This would mean far more patients on more statins, a situation that the NHS can't afford, so GP targets are likely to remain unchanged.

The vast majority of men in the UK, and a substantial minority of women, have an LDL above 1.81 mmol/l but most are at low risk of heart disease and shouldn't go anywhere near a statin. Alas, the aggressive promotion of the link between cholesterol and heart disease and the availability of over-the-counter statins has meant that a lot more lower-risk patients are taking drugs they don't need. A major study conducted among healthy Scots (yes, there are a few) found that if 10,000 people took statins for five years, 9,755 would receive no benefit. They would all, however, suffer from the medical dependency of lifelong medication and some would get unpleasant (and rarely, very serious) side effects.

Statins are of huge benefit to those at high risk of heart disease, and no use, or even harmful, to those at low risk. But, like blood pressure medicines, they only work if you take them for life and this is where it all starts to fall apart. The majority of patients on statins either stop taking the drug altogether or take less than the prescribed dose within a year. In the long-term, only a third of patients take them effectively. Instead of toughening up the targets and extending the net to create more cholesterol patients, we should concentrate our efforts on those at highest risk and make their tablet taking as simple, low-dose and side effect-free as possible. Of the £20 billion spent globally on statins, up to £14 billion could already be wasted on patients who refuse to take them. Surely not a time to prescribe more.

Reconfiguration

2 November 2006

Why has Labour failed to win the hearts and minds of doctors for its reform programme? For a while it won their silence, by stuffing their mouths with gold and cutting waiting times for surgery. But last week, in the fag end of Blair's administration, hundreds of members of the most politically apathetic profession donned catchy 'Working for a better NHS' scarves and marched on parliament, mumbling 'NHS SOS'.

There is a groundswell of opinion amongst doctors that the Government has badly screwed up its '£100 billion a year' chance to save the NHS, at least in England. Its biggest error has been to become so preoccupied with attracting private business that it has neglected to reconfigure the NHS until hospitals are deeply in debt. So even rational decisions about which hospitals and services need to close or merge for safety reasons are clouded in protests about finance and privatisation. Add in the political sensibilities of closures in marginal constituencies, and the most important reform is doomed to failure.

Since exposing the Bristol cardiac disaster in 1992, I have argued that specialist, hi-tech services have to be centralised in fewer centres where resources are concentrated and there is a sufficient caseload for safe training and meaningful audit. The *Eye* has exposed a succession of scandals where surgeons were doing highly complex operations occasionally, and often badly, and successfully campaigned for children's liver surgery and cleft palate repair to be restricted to fewer, accredited centres.

As technology has advanced over the last fifteen years, and the European working time directive kicked in, the centralisation argument has applied to more specialties. There are too many district general hospitals in the NHS and too many small casualty departments and paediatric units. This was evident when Labour took office and if they'd used the goodwill of the initial cash injection to get NHS staff and patients to agree on how local services needed to change, they might have succeeded.

Instead they threw the money at ill-conceived PFI deals, private surgical contractors, pointless quangos, the destruction of GP fundholding, the creation of 300 PCTs, the destruction of half of the PCTs and the reintroduction of GP fundholding. The attempt to introduce market competition and get money to follow the patient kicked off with a disastrous tariff system that didn't compensate hospitals for the risk and complexity of their work and led to record debts and the resignation of the chief executive, Nigel Crisp. The 2007–08 tariff has just been announced, and trusts will have to spend an enormous amount of time trying to 'unbundle it' (i.e. fight with each other to make sure they get paid for all their bits of treatment).

As in America, a hospital's survival will become entirely dependent on the success of its coding and debt collection departments, which are a hugely expensive, administrative cash drain. Contrast this to the tariff-free NHS in Scotland, which is well down the road of reconfiguration thanks to a clear national plan, extensive parliamentary debate, cross-party support and the involvement of staff and patients. Markets and fragmentation don't work in healthcare; consultation and co-operation do. Alas, it's too late for the English NHS.

NICE Rationing

12 December 2006

It's not often that a front-bench MP admits that rationing in the NHS exists, and has to exist, so hats off to shadow health secretaries Andrew Lansley (Con) and Steve Webb (Lib Dem). Admittedly I put the words in their mouths, but they repeated them without much prompting.

The occasion was the National Institute for Health and Clinical Excellence (NICE) conference, which I was paid to chair (though an assessment of my value for money is pending). Representing Labour was GP/MP Howard Stoate, who wouldn't admit to rationing but made up for it by declaring that the Government's reform programme was too quick and in the wrong order. Alas, he's unlikely to become health secretary.

NICE exists to try to make the rationing of healthcare rational. After lengthy analysis of the evidence, it approves most treatments but gets a good media kicking for taking its time to reach a judgement (Herceptin) or deciding which treatments shouldn't be funded by the NHS (Alzheimer's drugs in early dementia, Velcade for myeloma).

The result is a covert system of co-payments, where the rich top up their NHS treatment with private prescriptions for non-NICE approved drugs. This, according to Professor Karol Sikora, is happening throughout the NHS. So what's to stop cancer specialists offering private patients expensive new drugs that only add a few months to life? Their conscience, apparently.

But Labour's health reforms are not evaluated with the same rigour as new treatments. If Patsy Hewitt really wants to convince the public about NHS reconfiguration, she needs to publish detailed service planning and a rationale which can be supported by evidence. Alas, all she has is ideology. Crippling hospitals with PFI debts and throwing money at Independent Sector Treatment Centres (ISTCs) to cherry-pick easy operations has no evidence base, other than the splintered, debt-ridden service it has spawned.

The most compelling evidence that the health reforms have failed is that, under Blair, the gap between rich and poor has widened. The UK has one of the most unequal societies in Europe and every one of Labour's solutions has inadvertently made it worse. Waiting-list initiatives and patient-choice programmes favour the well-educated, who are also more likely to read and act on NICE guidelines. This isn't all Labour's fault; there's an inherent bias amongst NHS staff, especially doctors, to favour patients who are more like themselves.

In contrast, poorer patients are less likely to access good preventative care and routine surgery, and hence very reliant on the very emergency services which Labour are closing. The provision of healthcare has always been poor where the need is greatest, and excluding the obese and smokers from treatment, as is happening in some areas, will widen the gap further. Poorer patients often have more than one illness and the window of opportunity for treatment is narrow. If Labour was really concerned about equality, it would prioritise treatment on the basis of postcode so the poor get treated more quickly than the rich. And it would reinstate a properly funded public health specialty to evaluate its reforms. As Professor Rod Griffiths told the conference: 'The poor aren't "hard to reach". The tobacco industry and drug pushers have no problem reaching them. It's just that the politicians and the NHS don't want to.'

Expenses Update

Andrew Lansley spent more than £4,000 of taxpayers' money renovating his country home months before he sold it. He has repaid £2,600 of decorating fees.

Choose and Book Balls

26 December 2006

In September 2005, 78-year-old *Eye* reader Gordon Beare had a knee operation. This made one leg shorter than the other, necessitating orthopaedic shoes to level them up. Until recently, his GP would have organised referral to the orthotic department of his local hospital but under the new system of Choose and Book, Mr Beare has to organise his own referral by phoning up the Clinical Assessment Service (01296 710986 between 9.00 and 17.00 Monday to Friday excluding public holidays). He then has to choose one of fifteen units on offer and quote his unique booking reference number (0000–9236–9596) and unique computer-generated password ('cake counter').

If he prefers, he can book over the internet at www.nhs.uk/ healthspace and select 'choose and book'. However, he needs to be careful entering his password to put a space between 'cake' and 'counter'. If he doesn't like 'cake counter' he can go back to his GP and ask for it to be changed, or he can do it over the phone (0845 60 88 88 8), via text phone (0845 8 50 22 50) or internet (see above).

More important for Mr Beare is to know which of the fifteen units makes the best orthopaedic shoes but, alas, he is given no information as to the competence of the shoe-makers. He was also given no information about getting transport to and from any of the fifteen units, a pressing concern for someone with unequal legs. So, he phoned up and opted for his nearest unit (Colchester) who offered him a choice of two appointments six weeks apart, but was told to contact his GP about arranging transport.

His GP no longer arranges transport and he was given a number to ring (01206 742354) which he thinks might be an ambulance service but in any case couldn't offer him transport as he was outside of their area. As Mr Beare or Cake space Counter, as he is now known, puts it: 'Should I give up? Is it all a dream? At 78 I don't want all this aggro.'

Neither, it appears, do many doctors. GPs have an ethical and legal duty to refer patients to safe, high-quality services but neither they, nor their patients, are given any meaningful outcome data on which to base their choice. In the old system, consultants could prioritise patients referred to them, but under Choose and Book, it's up to the GP to prioritise the problem, which he or she may not feel able to do. An investigation by *Pulse* magazine found that electronic referrals do not always arrive in time for the appointment, or can't be opened, and that referral management centres are cancelling or diverting referrals deemed inappropriate.

Jeremy Fairbank, a consultant at the Nuffield Orthopaedic Centre NHS Trust, described the system as 'complex, expensive and unworkable.' Jonathan Edwards, a professor at University College London, is having 'every possible problem'. Dr Paul Reilly, a rheumatologist at Frimley Park Hospital in Surrey, claimed preferential treatment given to C&B patients meant 'trivial problems are seen ahead of serious ones.' And Dr Mark Pugh on the Isle of Wight has given up on the screening software as 'it is a pain in the arse to use.'

To be fair, some GPs, such as Labour MP Howard Stoate, positively enjoy using Choose and Book, but the over-complicated transfer of power and responsibility to patients without adequate information or engagement of doctors could lead to depersonalisation, discontent and disaster. And it's no way to get a pair of orthopaedic shoes.

Expenses Update

Howard Stoate has agreed to stop claiming a second home allowance as he only lives in Darford.

More GP Balls

26 January 2007

There are few sights less edifying in the NHS than Patricia Hewitt's brass neck, and it reached goitrous proportions with her latest attack on 'greedy, lazy' GPs. By committing the heinous crime of hitting all their targets and delivering precisely what their government-negotiated contract asked of them, they are guilty of bankrupting the NHS. Right.

Contrast this with the contracts offered to private companies to take over NHS diagnostics and surgery. These were guaranteed (i.e. paid whether patients were seen or not), paid above the going rate and allowed the cherry-picking of easy cases while leaving the NHS to mop up any cock-ups or act as a sink for patients too sick to turn a profit. Despite all these advantages, many companies have failed to treat their target volume of patients.

Doctors have also voiced concerns about the quality of care provided in Independent Sector Treatment Centres (ISTCs). This was dismissed by the Government as protectionist scaremongering but on the day Hewitt went for the GPs' jugular, the Healthcare Commission announced that the data on the clinical quality of ISTCs was 'incomplete and of extremely poor quality'. So what's the story? GPs fulfilling their contracts and collecting their payments, or expensive, unfair, under-performing and unaudited private treatment centres?

The healthy sums paid to GP partners were entirely predictable. Dangle a big carrot in front of intelligent, ambitious small businesses and it tends to get eaten. Unlike ISTCs, GPs have now contributed a huge amount of data to be entered into the NHS IT programme, should it ever deliver on its (under-performing, hugely overspent) contract. What's harder to assess is whether the GP contract will radically improve patient care and provide value for money. There are early signs that diabetic care is improving, and perhaps the care for patients with heart disease and stroke, but it's hard to prove because there was very little comparative data prior to the contract.[1]

Removing out-of-hours obligations from GPs and carving general practice up into targets is merely a way of introducing privatisation. The blame heaped on GPs for doing what was asked of them will further fuel the argument for more competition. Companies who have saturated the healthcare market in their own countries are using the NHS as a gateway to Europe, waved in by Labour. The Government recently published its NHS Operating Framework, which makes an interesting comparison to the ten core principles that they set out in the 2000 NHS Plan. Seven years ago, they pledged that 'Public funds for healthcare will be devoted solely to NHS patients.' This pledge has now been quietly shelved, as public funds for healthcare are increasingly devoted to the shareholders of private companies.

The latest game is to privatise outpatients by littering the country with Capture Assess Treat and Support (CATS) centres. Patients referred to hospital will be caught in Netcare's net whether they chose to be or not. White-elephant PFI-indebted hospitals won't be able to compete and will try to cannibalise surrounding hospitals, which are already running over capacity. And demand from an ageing population will rise year on year. The latest delusion is that transferring hospital services to GPs with special interests is cheaper (it isn't) and will reduce demand. The more you train GPs, the more they realise what is possible and the more they refer to hospital. The NHS is heading for meltdown and once again, it'll all be the GPs' fault.

---

[1] www.gpcontract.co.uk

Doctors Not To Be

8 March 2007

Are the careers of eight thousand junior doctors being stuffed up on purpose? The rushed implementation of the Modernising Medical Careers (MMC) programme looks like just another Labour cockup, but its consequences are suspiciously advantageous to a Government intent on busting the medical cabal.

The failure of the Medical Training Application Service (MTAS), a centrallycontrolled computerised bun fight, was predictable to anyone with a passing knowledge of NHS IT programmes. It was flawed in its content, an unvalidated bullshitters' paradise that has allowed erudite disaster zones to get jobs at the expense of much better doctors, and flawed in its delivery. Making so many doctors apply at the same time was bound to lead to persistent crashing of the site, lost applications, interviews offered for specialities not even applied for and interviews at both ends of the country on the same day.

The Government has been able to ignore earlier concerns that the new system was unfair and unworkable, safe in the knowledge that doctors are finding it hard to get public sympathy. Greedy GPs and consultants, rather than privatisation and target-chasing, have been cleverly fingered as the prime cause of NHS debt, and junior doctors bleating to the media that they may have to become lawyers, work in the City or move to Australia will have Patsy Hewitt chuckling in her cornflakes. The shit has finally reached the fan, thanks to West Midlands surgeons suspending their junior appointments, but health minister Lord Hunt was unfazed: 'MMC was devised with the help and support of the Royal Colleges, the Academy of Medical Sciences and the BMA.' So it's all their fault.

But what's in it for Labour? Having acknowledged they were stuffed by the BMA over consultant and GP contracts, the Government – having increased doctors' numbers – now wants to get by with as few as possible. Doctors have priced themselves out of the market, so medicine is being broken down into simplistic tasks that can be hived off to private companies employing lowest common denominator health workers. Having 30,000 junior doctors compete for 22,000 jobs creates sufficient anxiety and insecurity for those with a job to work illegal hours covering holes in the NHS without whistle-blowing.

Junior doctors aren't going down without a fight (support them at www.remedyuk.org) but is seems unlikely that enough would resign en masse to panic the Government. A more likely scenario is that they'll cancel their memberships of the BMA and Royal Colleges, a situation that would delight Labour. The GMC has already been stuffed by Liam Donaldson's ludicrously bureaucratic re-licensing plans, and taking out the rest of the medical establishment would make doctors even easier to control.

The Department of Health has announced a review of MTAS, but not suspended it. Thousands of juniors have joined up as Remedy UK, and are planning a protest on March 17 from the Royal College of Physicians to the Royal College of Surgeons. But to get public and media support, doctors need to explain how their personal misfortune will affect patients.

For the NHS to thrive, it has to ensure the best and brightest doctors are given the right jobs. MTAS doesn't appear capable of ensuring this. When I'm finally dragged kicking and screaming into an NHS ward, I want to be treated by a doctor with sufficient wisdom, skill and motivation to do the job properly, not a dumbed-down generic health worker reading from a guideline. Cutting down the supply of good doctors may well balance the NHS books in time to save Hewitt, but the long-term consequences will be dire for patient safety.

Cancer Jabs

22 March 2007

Have you taken your daughter for a cervical cancer jab yet? I've yet to be asked for it by any parent, but I know several doctors who've vaccinated their daughters against human papilloma virus types 16 and 18, which cause 70% of cervical cancers. One has vaccinated her sons too, on the back of a *Lancet* editorial that argued all adolescents should be immunised against HPV.[1] This would prevent men passing on these cancerous strains to unvaccinated women, and the vaccine (Gardasil) has the added bonus of protecting against HPV types 6 and 11, which cause 90% of genital warts. Having spent hours in a stuffy clinic trying to freeze them off, I'm sure this would be a huge bonus all round.

Not everyone agrees. Dr Angela Raffle, a public health specialist who oversees cervical screening in the Bristol area, described the editorial as 'disastrous for public health. Countries with high mortality and no screening can achieve major benefit from vaccination. But rushed implementation in Europe will undermine existing cervical screening – which already averts 80% of cervical cancer deaths – and leave women less protected than now.'[2]

True, girls who've been vaccinated might not bother to have cervical screening in later life. The vaccine only protects against 70% of cases of cervical cancer and it's not yet clear how long the protection lasts for. So cervical screening would still be needed to check the effectiveness of the vaccine and pick up the 30% of cancers that aren't covered. However, screening itself is no picnic – minor smear changes cause considerable anxiety and later stage pre-cancerous changes are unpleasant to treat with significant side effects.

[1] *Lancet* 7 October 2006.
[2] *Lancet* letters 3 February 2007.

If the vaccine works as well as the manufacturers (Sanofi Pasteur MSD) say it does, the side effects of screening would be greatly reduced since, as well as protecting against cancer, it should also reduce smear abnormalities at all stages. After the Vioxx scandal, some doctors are reluctant to trust data presented by MSD. But the safety and efficacy information have seen Gardasil get a licence in over 40 countries and it seems unlikely that an 'empty shell' vaccine, with no genetic viral material in it, could pose significant risks.

A bigger challenge is convincing the tabloids of the wisdom of vaccinating pre-teen girls and getting the cash-strapped NHS to foot the bill for a national immunisation plan. The immune response to the vaccine is better if it is given at an early age. No-one suggests that the rubella jab encourages girls to have sex, but the knowledge that cervical cancer is caused by a sexually transmitted infection has turned HPV vaccination into a red-top 'sex jab for schoolgirls'.

Immunisation programmes are up and running in the US, Australia and several European countries but Labour's plan to introduce immunisation for girls in their first year at secondary school looks like missing the boat this September. The decision was supposed to be announced in January, by the Joint Committee on Vaccination and Immunisation, but now seems destined to be delayed until at least June, too late to introduce for the start of the school year. This may just be traditional British scepticism, but the record NHS debts don't help and one DoH source has suggested Gordon Brown wants to make the announcement himself, on becoming a 'woman-friendly' twinkle-toothed premier. Quite how friendly this would be to girls who miss out on protection for the sake of political expediency is unclear. In the meantime, the vaccine is only available privately (£241.50 for three injections plus labour) or from a brave GP prepared to risk the wrath of the PCT.

Junior Doctor Job Fiasco (continued)

30 April 2007

Ever wanted to be a doctor? Couldn't get the grades? Well now you don't have to. Just log onto the MTAS website and you can access the personal details of hundreds of junior doctors. Why do medicine the hard way when you can become a doctor overnight with identity fraud?

This laughable security lapse in the on-line job application software for doctors and medical students has now been fixed . . . but only by taking down the whole site. So, with just thirteen weeks to go before August 1, junior doctors can't get any details of where and when their interviews are. But health minister Lord Hunt was wheeled out to assure us that 'top security advisers' from 'expert external companies' were looking at the lapses as a matter of urgency (and public cost).

Most disturbing was not the leaking of the sexual orientation and religion of named doctors (given the record of IT in the NHS, this was to be expected) but that such a spreadsheet existed in the first place. Such details should only ever be collected anonymously to ensure lack of discrimination, not attributed to named individuals when the only result can be to increase discrimination. So the Modernising Medical Careers programme may now face legal challenges for breaching confidentiality, as well as being incompetent and unfair.

Hunt tried to put the initial lapse down to a malicious leak, and then 'teething problems'. But when it emerged that junior doctors could easily hack into each other's job applications and change them if they so desired, it became apparent that the whole programme was unsafe. A suitably smug Richard Granger, head of the much derided Connecting for Health (CfH) programme, claimed if he'd been in charge of MTAS, such a breach would not have occurred. Channel 4 then discovered that the personal details (private addresses, phone numbers, e-mails, mobiles) of doctors attending a CfH conference were left up on its website for two weeks after the breach was reported and could still be obtained by Google-whack months later.

Hurrah for Heart Surgeons

On a brighter note, heart surgeons have shown the benefits of publishing sensitive data. Public disclosure of death rates began in 2001, after the Kennedy report on the deaths of child heart patients in Bristol. The death rate for coronary artery bypass graft (CABG) patients after public disclosure was significantly lower than it had been before, falling from 2.4% to 1.8% with no evidence that higher-risk patients were denied surgery.[1] The difference here is that grass-roots doctors are collecting data and sharing it with patients because they believe it to be the right thing to do. Whereas Connecting for Health, Modernising Medical Careers and much of the Blair health reforms are ill-conceived, rushed, top-down disasters that are forced on the front line without consultation or agreement. They funnel billions away from patients into the pockets of private companies and they don't work. Blair may claim after ten years that he's saved the NHS, but he won't be around on August 1 when those juniors who haven't given up are still scrabbling around for jobs, and patients are wondering if they'll ever see a doctor.

What Should Gordon Do?

15 June 2007
What should Gordon Brown do with the NHS? He may want to put his 'unique stamp' on it, but Blairites are working around

[1] Bridgewater et al. Has the publication of cardiac surgery outcome data been associated with changes in practice in Northwest England? *Heart* Jan. 2007; doi:10.1136/hrt.2006.106393

the clock to progress the market reforms beyond the point of no return. The great con of Blair's NHS was to preach the rhetoric of patient power whilst handing over control, and a vast sum of public money, to the private sector. To argue that this is not privatisation of the NHS is nonsense, but then Blair excelled at that.

The tipping point for the NHS will come if Labour pushes through its plans to outsource up to £64 billion worth of commissioning to multinational corporations such as United Health. This would suit Blair's friends at McKinsey, who can charge a fortune to the NHS for brokering the deals and also represent many of the US companies who stand to gain. At least one senior executive at McKinsey has a staff pass at the Department of Health. In return, Blair will have ample boot-filling opportunities in America.

In Blair's absence, Patsy Hewitt is rushing through his agenda before her exit, aided by David 'Nibbler' Nicholson, the surprise choice as NHS chief executive, who leapt up the shortlist after a meeting with Blairite health guru Professor Paul Corrigan. Nicholson in turn has appointed an NHS management team that is putting intense pressure on strategic health authorities and PCTs to outsource their commissioning. The idea that PCTs will retain ultimate control (and hence keep the NHS public) is a myth.

So what is Brown to do? Clearly a return to the Old Labour Stalinism of diktat by bureaucracy is impossible. And yet Blair's model is equally didactic, suggesting market competition is the only way forward and peppering it with promises of choice, when patients only get to choose what the Government (or United Health) wants them too. The junior doctor selection crisis is the most extreme example of this – thousands of doctors who have worked for seven years or more in the NHS are allowed only one choice of job, in many cases only specifying a region (e.g. Scotland) rather than a hospital unit.

Stalin invented the internal market, the Tories introduced it to the NHS and Blair is polishing it to imperfection.

The NHS works because it is a one-stop shop – once you're in it, you get all the care you need. Contrast this to America, where patients who have brain tumours removed are sent home the next day if the insurance package does not include continuing care. If American managed-care corporations unleash their 'expertise' on the NHS, only an American system can result. Profitable patients are cherry-picked while unprofitable patients are dumped.

Brown must reverse this without seeming to be Old Labour. The solution is to deliver what Blair and Hewitt have pretended to promise: 'a devolved NHS where 80% of the decisions are made locally'. Working in the NHS is like pulling people out of a river without bothering to look at who's pushing them in. If Labour really wants patients to get involved in shaping services, it has to move the money upstream and stop the dysfunctional schism between top-down marketing and local decision-making. Most NHS resources now go on managing chronic illness, and many patients manage themselves perfectly well for all but three hours a year, when they're hanging round the surgery or outpatient clinic. Tapping into this expertise and getting patients to help other patients in their communities is the best hope of stopping the log-jam downstream. The message is simple. Local partnerships between patients and NHS staff work, market reforms don't. But will Brown swallow it?

ALAN JOHNSON
June 2007–June 2009

Alan 'Postie' Johnson was a popular and non-confrontational health secretary, perhaps destined for greater things if he stops insisting he isn't up to the top job. In the meantime, he's off to the Home Office for what's left of New Labour, having largely succeeded in making the NHS very low key for the last two years. Unusually for a politician, he was pleased that so few of his speeches made the front pages. Meanwhile, power and managerial responsibility had quietly been devolved to Lord Darzi, who had hoped to pass it on to other doctors before he gave up the job in July 2009.

Johnson has a touch of Blair's affable persona and, like his former leader, a keen sense of political timing. The NHS is about to go pear-shaped as money gets diverted to pay off the banking crisis and more disasters like Mid Staffordshire will inevitably rise to the surface. However, whether the equally precarious home office is a sensible place from which to launch a leadership challenge remains to be seen.

PRIVATE EYE
Flash Darzi Saves the World

12 July 2007
New health secretary Alan Johnson's charm offensive on the NHS was delayed by the weather, but he seems to have cottoned on to the fact that you can't run an organisation of 1.3 million people from a box in Whitehall, part-time, while the great over-washed in Hull are demanding parity in flood defences with Sheffield.

So instead, it's up to junior heath minister Professor Ara Darzi, an Armenian born in Baghdad and trained in Ireland, to save the NHS part-time, in between minimally invasive robot-assisted surgery and a family. The Darzi review of the NHS in London lists a long line of previous reviews that made no difference to the vast inequalities in healthcare. But this time he's going to 'listen to Londoners, build a clinical consensus, provide evidence for the recommendations and work with the mayor and London boroughs.'

Alas, politicians need 'quick wins', which means not enough listening and too much change, too quickly. Johnson is already sounding quite the hypocrite, promising an end to top-down meddling in this new era of Brownian motion. Johnson also demonstrated his naivety by claiming the increase in life expectancy since the war was entirely due to the great scientific advances of the NHS, rather than largely due to economic and public health improvements.

Poor people get sick, and tackling poverty is a far better way of reducing health inequality than pouring money into the NHS. For those requiring NHS treatment, the biggest issue is the training and competence of the staff, rather than how healthcare is delivered (on the bus, in Tesco's, at a polyclinic). The front line of the NHS is very light on experience, and the generalists who can sort out the frail, obese elderly are a dying breed. Intensive care is full of 85-year-olds, slowly having the life sucked out of them and preventing further waiting-list reductions, and yet huge pressure is still piled on to hit the eighteen-week referral-to-treatment target. Less urgent patients leapfrog over the urgent every day. Johnson needs to give power for clinical decisions back to the staff, but will Brown be able to let go? Whatever happens, Darzi will survive. Anaesthetists often commit suicide because they have self-doubt and access to good drugs. Surgeons rarely do, because they are always right.

Child Ill-Health

20 August 2007

'There is now real concern and increasing evidence that the NHS is failing children.' So says Alan Craft, a professor of child health in Newcastle, in a *BMJ* editorial (August 11, 2007). This despite Labour's 'National Service Framework for Children', belatedly launched in 2004 in response to the Bristol scandal.

Alas, children don't vote and they tend not to take to the streets to complain about their care, so there was no additional money or specific targets for Labour's vision. Last year, the Healthcare Commission found that only 4% of trusts had made excellent progress in implementing the framework, and 21% rated good. Most progress was made in 'improving the hospital environment' but there was still 'a worrying potential for unsafe medical care'. That is, surgeons trained to operate on adults are still operating on children too, many on just a handful a year, making their results statistically meaningless.

Recruitment into high-risk, high-litigation paediatric specialties remains a problem and the service trundles on, with some hospitals lacking the staff to provide life support for children during the day and one in five unable to deal effectively with paediatric emergencies at night. The alternative, to close smaller units and merge services on fewer, bigger sites is politically unpalatable and they may still be unable to cope with the workload.

Good paediatric services are vital to the future of the NHS and without them the burden of chronic illness into adulthood is huge. The damage of passive smoking in pubs is negligible compared to the damage to a child if a mother smoked during pregnancy. If you survive your small, shrivelled placenta *in utero*, your risks of heart disease and premature death as an adult are greatly increased. I have written previously about the importance of fluoride for dental health, folic acid to prevent spina bifida and neonatal hearing tests to pick up deafness early, and yet the UK still has a lamentably poor record in preventative health for babies and children.

The UK also has one of the highest incidences of childhood diabetes and worst records of diabetic control, but the long-term devastation this causes is beyond the scope of short-term political targets. Our detection and survival rates for childhood cancer are amongst the worst in Europe and we're fifteenth in the European league table for perinatal mortality.

For the NHS to survive, it needs to invest in keeping children healthy upstream to prevent a log-jam later on. Programmes like Sure_Start and improvements in community child mental health services are starting to kick in but good hospital treatment is being stifled by targets for adult surgery and waiting times, as well as the difficulties in setting a fair tariff for complex paediatric care that requires input from many specialties. In a market NHS, paediatric care will only flourish if it can turn a profit. At present, much of it is cheap, unsafe and done on the hoof by non-specialists. Brown and Johnson need to refocus away from markets and back onto quality and safety.

Lord Darzi's Balls

4 October 2007

Who'd be Professor the Lord Darzi of Denham (FREng, KBE, FMedSci)? When asked by John Humphrys on the *Today* programme why his NHS review would be any different to any of the previous NHS reviews, he said 'Ee ah ah um colleagues.' He then trotted out the 'envy of the world' homily before being reminded that the NHS ranked seventeenth (out of 29) in the latest league table of European healthcare (behind Latvia). So should the NHS consider some level of charging? 'Governments will have to look at that in more clearly.' Eh?

No matter, there was still the hard copy of *Our NHS Our Future: NHS Next Stage Review Interim Report October 2007* to wade through. I hope this was rushed out as a cynical piece of electioneering. Otherwise, there's no excuse for 'we now need to change the way we lead change – effective change needs to be animated by the needs and preferences of patients, empowered to make their decisions count within the NHS with the response to patients' needs and choices being led by clinicians taking account of the best available evidence.'

I've never met a surgeon who speaks like that. Has Lord Darzi's brain been replaced with Labour arse gravy? 'Patients can feel like a number, rather than a person.' Hardly surprising when Choose and Book reduces you to a unique 12-digit PIN along with easy-to-remember computer-generated password ('fountain saver', 'broccoli spot', 'cake counter'). But the most striking claim is that the review 'is not about changing the way the NHS is structured'. So what is merging specialist services onto fewer sites, merging GPs into 'federated polyclinics' and downsizing district general hospitals?

Darzi has joined the party halfway through, when so much money has already been wasted on NHS change that he'll have a job convincing the staff of the need for more. He's proposing polyclinics to do much of the work done in district general hospitals, but we've already invested £1.4 billion in Independent Sector Treatment Centres that were supposed to do the same. ISTCs were encouraged into the market with guaranteed contracts paid above tariff. Last year, they were paid for 50,000 more operations than they carried out. The vast majority of waiting-list reductions were carried out in existing NHS hospitals and a huge sum has been wasted on unnecessary competition.

The NHS already has a competitive market under Payment By Results. Or rather activity. Hospitals can only survive by sucking as many patients as possible through their doors. ISTCs couldn't attract the custom, not least because they failed to submit sufficient outcome information to the Healthcare Commission to enable them to be audited for quality and safety.

Polyclinics may well have the expertise to treat patients closer to home but whether they can stand up to the might of desperate hospitals remains to be seen. To get the support of NHS staff, Darzi doesn't just need to consult them, he needs to publish evidence showing his reforms would work. The Academy of Medical Royal Colleges has performed the most comprehensive review of the reconfiguration plans and agrees that highly specialised services such as major trauma, heart and brain surgery need to be specialised on fewer sites. But it found no evidence to support the centralisation of the non-complex, high-volume work done in district general hospitals.

There is, however, evidence that patients feel access to GPs has improved in the last few years, which makes Brown and Darzi's peculiar focus on extending opening hours puzzling. The review smells strongly of hastily assembled populist opinion. Clinical medicine has been reformed in the last twenty years by focusing on the evidence, not the expert. The same needs to happen with NHS reform. Don't change the system until you can prove you've got something better.

Denying the Dying

14 November 2007

'What's the point of giving millions to cancer charities and spending billions on developing new drugs, often in the UK, if the NHS won't pay for them?' So asks Graham Smith, whose junior doctor son Ollie died from metastatic colon cancer at the age of 29, and who was denied the drug Avastin (bevacizumab) by Harrow PCT. The PCT was following guidance from NICE, which in January 2007 decided that Avastin did not represent a good enough use of NHS funds.

Strange, then, that it should be available across Europe and America. Avastin is a genetically engineered version of a mouse antibody that contains both human and mouse components. It is believed to work by inhibiting a protein that stimulates new blood vessels, thus denying tumors blood, oxygen and other nutrients needed for growth.

It is not a cure for metastatic cancer, but got its FDA licence in America in 2004 for use alongside chemotherapy because it 'has been proven to delay tumor growth and more importantly, significantly extend the lives of patients'. This may only be by a matter of months, but it can also extend the disease-free survival and so patients and relatives may be spared some of the relentless decline of metastatic cancer which transformed Ollie from 'a handsome fit young man to a grotesquely deformed blind and crippled old man in twelve weeks'.

Expensive as Avastin is (£2,500 per infusion), drug costs constitute a very small fraction of the overall cost to the NHS of treating cancer, with most resources spent in the last few months of life. If a drug keeps a patient out of hospital for longer, it could easily justify its cost. Roche, who manufacture the drug with Genentech, also make Herceptin and have a licence for Avastin in metastatic lung and breast cancer. Trials are ongoing to see if the drug works in early-stage cancers, where it has a better chance of cure, and the results are likely to lead to another lengthy bout of NICE deliberation. Roche has thus far played hardball with the price, arguing that it took over 30 years of research to find a monoclonal antibody able to delay tumour growth. They also believe the drug is worth the money, and that sufficient individuals and insurers will fork out, even if the NHS doesn't.

In May this year, the influential (and independent) Karolinska Institute in Sweden found that the 'excessive bureaucracy' involved in approving drugs for use (or not) in the NHS was one reason for our higher death rates. However, other European countries are looking at the NICE model as a way of containing their own drug costs and many also adopt its guidance.

All of which puts doctors in a difficult position. According to his father, Ollie's oncologist strongly recommended the use of Avastin in his treatment and thought the NHS would provide it. It was unanimously denied by the PCT initially and on appeal because of 'the duty to balance the needs of the individual with the needs of the wider population'. Had Ollie decided to take to the streets *à la* Herceptin ('young, handsome junior doctor who has given his life to caring for the sick denied vital cancer drug') he would doubtless have got it. Colon cancer in someone so young is rare, and its detection was doubtless delayed because of the long hours and hectic lifestyle of a trainee surgeon. Two doctors advised him he had irritable bowel syndrome.

Ollie's only demand was for his parents to reunite so he could die at home. His father remains incredulous that he was denied a licensed treatment, available in most other European countries. Living a few more months with a better quality of life doesn't sound like much until you try without.

Conflict of Interest: I have been paid to chair conferences for NICE and Roche. My views remain somewhere between the two.

In Praise of Bolton

1 February 2008
'By 2008, no-one will have to wait longer than eighteen weeks from GP referral to hospital treatment.' So said Labour's NHS Improvement Plan in June 2004. The definition of 'by 2008' is a little blurred. The key targets are that by March, 85% of patients needing hospital admission and 90% of those who don't should have a 'referral to treatment' time of eighteen weeks or less. It isn't until the end of December that it applies to all patients (but only if they want it to).

The 18-week website (www.18weeks.nhs.uk) has a helpful clock in the top left-hand corner (333 days to go!), but many PCTs are in despair about how to do it. 'Diagnostics' presents a particular challenge. When the target was announced, the waiting time in many areas for MRI scans was two years, but Bolton PCT has somehow managed to get the wait down for all diagnostic tests (apart from the odd six-week endoscopy) to two weeks.

So how's it done? Bolton PCT has some experienced, workaholic and ballsy commissioners who were reasonably solvent when they started planning in 2005. Some of their solutions were obvious (getting Royal Bolton Hospital's imaging department to stay open over lunch), others were inspired (instead of pissing off all the consultants by parking a private scanner in the hospital car park, they took it into the community). They gave GPs direct access to urgent community scans for patients with abdominal pain and breathlessness, so they didn't have to be sent to A&E, kept in overnight and often not discharged for several days.

The growth of community scanning has forced the hospital to improve its service and the PCT can now insist that scans are reported on within four days (often sooner) with a treatment plan that the GP and patients can understand. And they're developing an IT system that allows the scans to be whizzed from hospital or scanner to GP surgery. By December 2007, 99% of patients who didn't need to be hospitalised were treated within eighteen weeks as were 92% of those who did.

Bolton is not the healthiest place to live – the life expectancy is several years less than, say, Dorset – but the fact that a deprived area has achieved such improvement when much of the rest of the NHS (particularly in the south) is still riven by petty, internecine, inter-professional rivalries is extraordinary.

Faster access to diagnostic tests is not a panacea. It's expensive, it encourages doctors to reach for the scanner rather than examine patients, it requires considerable operator skill, there is no mandatory regulation of the sonographers who perform ultrasounds, it throws up anxiety-provoking false results and it can increase exposure to unnecessary radiation. And under the old 'watch and wait' NHS rationing, some patients got better (or gave up) on their own. However, used correctly, a good scan will pick up your cancer, heart failure or leaking aneurysm far more quickly than if you sat at home waiting for the PCT and hospital to finish squabbling over who should be doing the scanning. So well done Bolton. Lord Darzi should pay them a visit.

Letter of the Week

15 February 2008

Sir,

I received Alan Johnson's letter today 'Improving access to GP services', and having just seen my last patient, I read it and thought I'd respond by phone. His number is on the letter. I spoke to a very nice chap and explained that having received Mr Johnson's letter there were a couple of things I'd like to discuss with him. He asked me to hold and then came back on the line to say that Mr Johnson wasn't available, and in fact there was no one at all at the DoH who could discuss this letter with me, as they all go home by 5pm.

I'm delighted that at least everyone at the DoH finishes early enough to be able to see their own GP in a normal evening surgery without the need for extended opening hours.

Paul Baird
Portesham Surgery
Weymouth

Patient McChoice

21 March 2008

'The Good Hospital Guide. From Cardio to Cancer – where to get the best treatment.' So proclaims the front page of the *Independent* (March 20), to coincide with Labour's April 1 pledge that patients requiring non-emergency treatment can travel to any NHS hospital in England, or indeed any private one that has an NHS contract. Alas, the *Indy*'s extensive guide lists just ten 'best' hospitals, all in London. For 'eyes' it recommends Moorfields Hospital, whose latest Healthcare Commission rating for quality of services was 'weak', and for 'bones and joints' it goes for the Royal National Orthopaedic Hospital in Stanmore (HC rating, 'fair'). The Royal Marsden Hospital for cancer does at least have an 'excellent' rating but 'cancer is one of the specialties excluded from the extended patient choice agenda.'

The *Indy*'s sparse recommendations are entirely based on reputation, but patient choice is pointless without outcome data that provides a meaningful comparison between different centres for each specific treatment. How likely is it that the treatment will improve my quality of life? How likely is it that it will kill or maim me? The Government and NHS have been painfully slow to roll this information out for other specialties, but BUPA has been collecting patient-reported outcome measures (PROMs) since 1999, in the wake of the carnage caused by rogue gynaecologist Rodney 'the butcher' Ledward. Patients complete a standardised questionnaire (e.g. EQ–5D available at www.euroqol.org) and are followed up at three and six months after surgery. Prospective patients can then be given a fair indication of how likely a treatment is to improve quality of life rather than just providing a pathology specimen and a six-inch scar.

The NHS is only now dabbling with PROMs, limiting

them to hernias, varicose veins and hip and knee replacements for 2008–09. This is a tacit acceptance that information gathering for BUPA (with largely middle-class, articulate, motivated patients) may be easier than following up NHS patients. A 70% response rate will require a huge amount of effort and my guess is that it will be dumped on GPs, who will refuse to do it.

In the meantime, patient choice will continue to be cosmetic and insubstantial. Hospitals can take on the most inappropriate corporate sponsors (some, such as Guy's, have had a McDonalds on site for years) and use their expertise to advertise services (but not directly discredit the services of their rivals). They can also enlist the help of celebrities who've been patients to publicly endorse the treatment they've received. Those who don't already jump the queue for a private room will be able to enhance their treatment with the promise of a free plug.

Most patients will choose to stick with their nearest hospitals but choice has the potential to improve quality and safety in the NHS by putting reliable, independent, unbiased performance data in the public domain and making all hospitals up their game. In contrast, adverts, sponsorship and celebrity endorsement will just be a breeding ground for yet more bias and spin.

The Politics of Prostate Cancer

10 April 2008

Why are men with early prostate cancer still being denied NICE-approved treatment? The disease kills ten thousand men a year, but the cancer is difficult to predict. In some it spreads rapidly and often presents too late for a cure, in others it remains localised in the prostate gland without causing any obvious harm. For the latter, radical surgery or radiotherapy may do more harm than good.

The research challenge is to develop better screening tests and identify those early cancers that are likely to spread. More localised treatments, which eradicate the cancer while sparing patients the misery of incontinence and impotence, are also needed. Brachytherapy, which inserts radioactive seeds into the prostate, is one such treatment for early cancer, and achieves as good a control of the disease as radical surgery with far fewer side effects. Indeed, it is the only minimally invasive treatment for the disease that is approved by NICE (February 2008).

This should, in theory, give a much better choice for men who decide they want to be tested for the disease and are found to have localised cancer. They can either choose to have surveillance rather than treatment, with the option of doing something later if the cancer starts to grow (NICE's preferred and cheapest option). Or they can choose to go straight for treatment, preferably with the fewest side effects. Brachy-therapy became available in the UK a decade ago, but many patients have been denied funding for it on the NHS. There was a blanket ban on all new NHS referrals from Wales between October 2005 and February 2007, and men are still being denied treatment despite NICE approval.

Others have taken on their PCT and won. Roy Stainton is a retired professor of operational mathematics who was found to have localised prostate cancer in 2004. His consultant at Winchester Hospital gave him a 'prostate cancer treatment toolkit' to mull over, but tried to remove the section on brachy-therapy because 'the PCT will never fund it.' Mr Stainton decided he wanted it and was swiftly declined.

Appealing against South Hants PCT wasn't easy. His GP knew very little about brachytherapy and he was left alone to assemble his case. He read up on the research, used it to inform his case, gathered letters of support and lodged his appeal. He was offered a hearing and the chance to respond to contrary evidence by the end of the day on which the letter arrived. He quickly reviewed the evidence and delivered his response by hand. He was also invited to take a medical representative with him, which he didn't have, and although the nice lady from the Patient Advocacy Liaison Service was keen, she didn't know anything about brachytherapy either.

At the hearing, the PCT mislaid his supplementary evidence, which was subsequently photocopied and circulated. Mr Stainton's statistical analysis showed that, when all convalescence costs were considered, brachytherapy was no more expensive than radical surgery, and cheaper in the long-term if side effects were avoided. Labour would no doubt claim this was patient advocacy in action. In reality, you're on your own and it helps if you're a statistical genius.

For every successful appeal, there are many more losers. Men are remortgaging their houses and going to small private clinics rather than larger specialist centres with the expertise to do brachytherapy properly.[1] The NICE guidance should finally end this, and make high-quality treatment available to all who choose it, but don't hold your breath.

Bring Back Safety First

8 May 2008

'I want to help use Elaine's death to help bring cultural change in healthcare. I want to tell our two young children when they have grown up that Mummy's death has made a big difference.' So says inspirational pilot Martin Bromiley on the website for his charity founded to recognise the role of human factors in the prevention of medical error (www.chfg.org).

---

[1] http://www.prostatebrachytherapyinfo.net/

Elaine Bromiley was 37 and healthy when she was booked in for non-emergency sinus surgery under general anaesthesia in a private unit adjacent to an NHS hospital. Her consultant anaesthetist had sixteen years of experience, the ENT surgeon had 30 years under his belt, and three of the four nurses in the theatre were also very experienced. The theatre was very well equipped, there were no competing pressures of emergencies elsewhere, but there was another senior anaesthetist operating in the theatre next door. As Bromiley observed: 'This was a dream scenario for safety. A senior, competent surgical team working in state-of-the-art surroundings.'

Anaesthesia was induced at 08.35 but it was not possible to insert the laryngeal mask airway. By 08.37, oxygenation began to deteriorate and she looked cyanosed. Her oxygen saturation dropped to 75% (anything below 90% is significantly low). By 08.39, oxygen saturation had fallen to 40% but attempts to ventilate the lungs with 100% oxygen using a facemask and oral airway proved extremely difficult. The saturation level remained perilously low but the anaesthetist, who was joined by a consultant colleague, was unable to perform a tracheal intubation.

By 08.45, airway access had still not been achieved and the situation was termed 'can't intubate, can't ventilate', a recognised emergency for which guidelines (requiring an emergency tracheotomy to establish an airway through the front of the neck) were well known. One nurse, on her own initiative, fetched the tracheotomy tray. Another, recognising the severity of the situation, went to secure a bed on the intensive care unit. However, the three consultants decided to keep attempting intubation, unsuccessfully, and at 09.10 abandoned the procedure hoping she would wake up. Her oxygen saturation had remained at less than 40% for twenty minutes and she never recovered consciousness, dying thirteen days later.

Martin Bromiley was initially told that his wife's death was extreme bad luck and that nothing more could have been done. As a pilot, he was used to analysing critical incidents in a no-blame culture and wanted to hear the results of the ensuing inquiry. He was told: 'There won't be an inquiry. Not unless you complain or sue.' Bromiley insisted on an independent expert review, which concluded that, given the skill mix of the clinicians, it should have been very easy to follow the established emergency protocol and perform a tracheotomy. So why didn't it happen?

Errors in medicine happen not just because of lack of skill or knowledge but for behavioural reasons. Ask doctors what they should do in an exam, and they trot out the guidelines. Put them in the extremely stressful situation of a very rare, rapidly deteriorating potential catastrophe and even the most senior clinicians can lose the plot. The role of these human factors in decision-making is well recognised in aviation and it is to his enormous credit that Bromiley has assembled leaders in the field to work out how such disasters can be prevented. Simulating emergency situations, pre-briefing and debriefing before surgery, introducing and valuing members of the team and creating a culture where the most junior member of staff (or even the patient) can raise concerns or call for a time-out sound obvious, but don't happen routinely in the NHS. And the drive for productivity and cost-containment under Labour is leading to yet more corner-cutting. For the sake of Elaine Bromiley, and the thousands of others who die each year from avoidable error, Lord Darzi's review must rebuild the NHS around safety.

Why Children Still Die

6 June 2008

Why Children Die, a detailed analysis of UK childhood death in 2006 (and published last month), has concluded that in 69% of deaths, there were avoidable or potentially avoidable factors. Equally alarming for a report that should be central to the reform of the NHS is that it has received virtually no publicity.

In the study, carried out by the Confidential Enquiry into Maternal and Child Health (CEMACH) with funding from the National Patient Safety Agency (NPSA), data was gathered on 957 deaths of children in three English regions, Wales and Northern Ireland. An expert panel examined 119 deaths in detail but the 'headline result of the panel data' is hidden away on page 47. According to one panel member, the release of the report was delayed by Labour citing purdah and neutered in response to pressure from the Cabinet Office and the Department of Health.

So what has the Government got to be frightened of? Despite a succession of declarations on patient safety, such as *An Organisation with a Memory*, and a large safety conference attended by Gordon Brown last month, the NHS appears not to be learning much from either the Bristol or Climbie disasters. In both medical and social care, children are still not getting access to expertise quickly enough. The recurring patterns of substandard care are depressingly familiar: poor care of sick children by staff not adequately trained in paediatrics or supervised by those who are; failure to recognise a sick/vulnerable child; failure of follow-up; failure to immunise; failure to refer to mental health services. Some of the findings were unexpected (e.g. high rates of child suicide), but avoidable factors related to clinical and organisational care were far more predictable and possibly made worse by the Government's reforms.

The devolution of frontline NHS care to the least experienced (and cheapest) staff is commonplace and 'in 8% of hospital trusts, surgeons carrying out elective surgery did not perform enough work with children to maintain their skills.' So why are strategic health authorities, commissioners and trusts allowing them to do it? Because trusts need the money and no-one is brave enough to enforce safety standards. And the current obsession with public involvement is cementing the future of small, inadequately staffed paediatric units serving similar maternity units. The public (and politicians) love a cosy local unit but no-one has the balls to tell them that lives are at risk when emergencies are badly managed.

The obsession with performance targets has meant many children have been erased from outpatient clinics if they fail to attend but trusts are making no attempt to detect those most at risk (who are hardly to blame if an adult forgets or isn't able to take them to hospital). Many operational policies and pathways still don't reflect best practice, referrals to the Coroner's office are still not managed properly and death certificates are still littered with errors.

On a brighter note, there were plenty of examples of excellent practice but, as ever, the NHS hopes that good care will spread by some mysterious osmosis from beacon sites rather than building reform from the bottom up on quality and safety. As of April, Local Safeguarding Children Boards have been set up to continue studying child deaths, but their current methodology (looking at unexpected deaths) will not identify all avoidable factors outlined in this excellent CEMACH study. There are salutary lessons here for everyone who works in (and uses) the NHS, but the fact that I only heard of *Why Children Die*[1] from a concerned *Eye* reader reveals how far Labour has to go before being open about the true extent of medical error.

[1] *Why Children Die.* CEMACH 2008. ISBN 978-0-9558055-0-9.

Darzi's Déjà Vu Review

1 July 2008

Will Lord Darzi be following Raj Persaud to the GMC on charges of plagiarism? His NHS review, *High Quality Care For All* (June 30, 2008), is alarmingly similar to Frank Dobson's 1998 bestseller, *A First Class Service: Quality in the New NHS.* Dobson's foreword starts: 'All patients in the National Health Service are entitled to high quality care', and promises that 'unacceptable variations that have grown up in recent years must end.' Just ten years later, Darzi stresses that tackling significant variations in the quality of care will be his first priority.

Dobson's reforms would ensure 'high quality care becomes the norm everywhere.' Darzi, in contrast, will deliver 'high quality for users of services in all aspects, not just some.' Dobson manages 191 mentions of 'quality' in his document compared to Darzi's 359. But Dobson put quality in every chapter heading (Setting Quality Standards, Delivering Quality Standards, Monitoring Quality Standards and Action for Quality.) So the claim that the Darzi review is radically different for its focus on quality is clearly bollocks.

Dobson put his paper out for consultation but Darzi has already consulted over 2,000 doctors and the fact that so many put variation in quality at the top of their agenda a decade after Labour promised to abolish it is frankly disturbing. In his foreword, Brown desperately tries to rewrite history by claiming that the first ten years of Labour were all about building capacity to get waiting lists down, and now it's time to focus on, um, quality. Perhaps he was sulking when Dobson tried just that.

There are lots of other similarities – promises to put patients at the centre of care, gather their opinions and give them outcome figures – but two key differences. Dobson's log made not a single mention of the word 'choice'. Darzi gives us 62 to choose from. Dobson is Old Labour, believes in co-operation in healthcare (along with the Scottish and Welsh assemblies) and that people don't want to shop around for treatment when they're ill. Blair quickly got rid of him and brought in Milburn to feed the NHS to the market. Lots of money, duplication and job insecurity has indeed got waiting lists down, but because the publication of clinical outcomes promised by Dobson and Milburn has never materialised, we still don't know if the onslaught on waiting lists will come at the price of failed cataract surgery and joint replacements later on. Quicker does not always mean better.

Dobson also believed that the healthy competition of professionalism would raise standards but Darzi has swallowed the Blair belief that staff need financial incentives to practise good care. So as well as reminding them to treat patients with dignity and respect (doh!), they will be paid extra for providing a 'new' quality service based on outcomes. Could this be an extension of the quality and outcomes framework that 'incentivised' GPs so well? Incentives work by undermining the neutrality of professional judgement and encouraging self-interested decision-making. They wouldn't be needed if good information on outcomes was published.

So, has the fag end of Labour got the stomach to do what it promised a decade ago? I first called for heart surgeons to publish their results back in 1992 and now they are doing so, but no-one else is. In 2001, the Paediatric Cardiac Services Review that followed the Kennedy inquiry recommended the number of units performing child heart surgery be reduced from thirteen to six to ensure quality and safety. There are still thirteen, because putting babies at risk is trumped by the political risk of closing a local service. On July 18, 2001, Alan Milburn promised in the Commons he would publish 'information for patients, and specifically for parents, before consenting to treatment for themselves or their children.' To date it has not appeared. If the last 60 years has taught us anything about the NHS, it's that – Nye Bevan aside – politicians can't deliver the hard stuff. Don't give up the day job, Darzi.

Not Warts and All

16 July 2008

Why has Labour chosen not to protect girls from genital warts as well as cervical cancer? I have written previously about the UK's delay in instigating a vaccination programme with Gardasil, which gives excellent protection against both diseases and has been widely used for over a year in the US, Canada, Australia and many European countries. Not only has the UK delayed introduction – presumably for cost reasons – but it has plumped for a cheaper vaccine, Cervarix, which only protects against cervical cancer.

Those unsure of how unpleasant warts can be should take a peek at http://www.chestersexualhealth.co.uk/genitalwarts.htm. Be warned – it isn't for the squeamish. I've worked in a sexual clinic and seen the devastation that warts cause to people's sex lives (often non-existent) and emotional well-being (sometimes profoundly depressed). They're extremely common, with upwards of 85,000 cases a year in England and Wales, costing £25 million annually to treat. There would have been a significant reduction in wart workload and anguish within a few years had Gardasil been chosen, and in time, the savings would easily compensate for the disparity in price between the two vaccines.

Labour's decision makes no economic, clinical or humane sense. On January 16, a letter from health secretary Alan Johnson to Colm O'Mahony, a sexual health consultant, suggests that Labour were at that stage opting for Gardasil: 'It is expected the vaccination of girls will reduce the transmission of infection to boys, by herd immunity, and reduce the number of genital warts cases in boys as well as girls.' So why the change of mind? Labour spouts all this guff about respecting and understanding patients and then makes an absurdly unempathic decision.

Johnson's prevarication over top-up payments centres on his dislike of two-tier health systems, but every sexual health consultant and GP I've spoken to is advising parents who can afford it to pay for Gardasil (£250 for three injections). Why would you not protect your daughter against warts if you could? Some doctors have had their sons vaccinated too. Warts can kill your sex life, treatment can be embarrassing and uncomfortable, and in a third of people they keep coming back.

Perhaps the market reforms of the NHS have left it so bankrupt that there simply isn't enough spare cash to fund the more expensive vaccine. But given that foundation hospitals have made record savings and are sitting on over £1 billion of taxpayers' money, this doesn't stack up. Labour – 'the champions of choice' – are denying parents the right to choose whether to protect their daughters against what can be a psychologically devastating, chronic infection. At the very least, those parents whose daughters are due to join the cervical cancer vaccination programme and want them to have the extra protection should be allowed to pay the difference between the two vaccines, rather than pay the whole cost of Gardasil. This is one top-up that's worth it.

Dr Phil's Notes

In Australia, they've offered Gardasil to 12-18 year old girls in a school-based program from April 2007, and it's also widely available to those not in school. By the end of 2008, researchers at the county's largest sexual health centre in Melbourne found a 48% decrease in genital warts in women aged under 28 years, saving a lot of money and anguish. However, they are worried that attempts to reduce genital warts will be undermined by backpackers from countries like the UK which do not vaccinate against them. I couldn't get Gardasil on the NHS and I wasn't allowed to top up so I bought it privately and gave it to my daughter myself. So strike me off.

Market Balls

1 August 2008

The key to the success of Lord Darzi's next-stage review is to 'put clinicians back in the driving seat' of the NHS. But do they understand where they're going? The service is now riddled with jargon invented by management consultants to justify their fee, and very few doctors have a clue what it means. Additionality. Contestibility. Service Line Reporting. Patient Level Activity Based Costing Solutions. Directed Enhanced Services. Extended Choice Network. Healthcare Resource Group version 4. Market Forces Factor. Secondary Users' Services. Unbundling the Tariff.

The situation is so dire that this year's Audit and Healthcare Commission report on Labour's reforms, *Is the Treatment Working?*, had to include a five-page glossary. Unsurprisingly, the report concluded there is no evidence that the imposition of choice and competition is improving the service. The Healthcare Commission's reward is to disappear up the arse of the new Care Quality Commission, where it will find it much harder to cause trouble.

According to the *Health Service Journal* (July 24), GPs keen on getting involved in practice-based commissioning (whatever that is) are not communicating well with PCTs when submitting 'service redesign bids'. So to help them write their business plans, everyone's favourite health minister Ben Bradshaw is bringing in more management consultants 'to establish a framework contract providing quality assured development support'.

Occasionally, doctors understand only too well what managers are getting at. The *HSJ* also reported a 'brutal culling' at Avon and Wiltshire Mental Health Trust, which has decided to replace its medical director (i.e. a doctor trying her hand at management), along with the finance director, while asking four other managers to reapply for their roles. I have now been sent the eight-page advert for the new combined role of medical director and director of strategy and business development.

The trust is looking for a doctor to 'drive the business development strategy in line with the Business Proposition, scanning the mental health environment for new opportunities and identifying and stimulating new business solutions that fit with the corporate vision'. The ad mentions 'profitability' four times. We no longer treat the mentally ill according to need. We have to make money out of them.

I have also been sent a draft contract between Dr Foster Research, the private company making millions out of (our) NHS data and drug-giant Pfizer. The contract is for a 'customised version of the population health manager tool' for £375,000 plus VAT. The tool uses NHS data to allow analysis of 'market sizing, hospital market share, GP referral patterns, benchmarking provider performance and understanding admission rates'. This will allow Pfizer to 'focus marketing and awareness-raising activity to stimulate growth'.

Labour's reforms can't succeed because, despite all Darzi's rhetoric of 'engagement', you can only unite the NHS around common values, and the emphasis on commodity and profitability is repugnant to many frontline staff. Labour can try to disguise its agenda through the bullshit of marketisation, but it still smells terrible.

Dangerous Surgery (No. 467)

29 August 2008

What's the definition of dangerous surgery? When you do the wrong thing (turn up pissed, cut off the wrong leg), it's obvious. But what if a surgical team attempts the correct procedure, but the patients keep dying? If you analyse each unexpected death (which doesn't always happen), you may spot something in the process of the operation (e.g. the surgeon was very slow) that might identify the problem. But for major surgery, a certain number of patients will die even in the best hands, and often it will take a number of operations for a pattern to emerge. Here, you need a statistical definition of danger to tell you that you are significantly worse at a particular operation than the average surgical team in the NHS, and you should stop operating and investigate.

That's the theory, but sixteen years after the *Eye* exposed the comparatively dangerous results for complex child heart surgery in Bristol, neither the Department of Health nor the Royal College of Surgeons has introduced such a statistical benchmark and, as a result, dangerous surgery still flourishes in the NHS. The General Medical Council covered its arse in 1998 by disciplining the Bristol surgeons for failing to act on their poor results, but the judgement was nonsensical without a statistical definition of poor. Without such a benchmark, you don't know when to stop.

The subsequent Public Inquiry nearly got there by spotting that a baby's overall chance of dying after complex heart surgery in Bristol between 1991 and 1995 was double the average rate in all the other NHS units. 'Double-the-average-mortality-elsewhere' should have been adopted as the danger benchmark across a whole range of major surgery where death is a significant risk. It would also require a surgical unit to prove its safety by doing enough of a particular operation to provide statistically significant results, and to carefully code and count each procedure to ensure the data was accurate.

Researchers at St George's Hospital in London have used this standard to analyse the repair of abdominal aortic aneurysms (AAA) in England between 2001 and 2005.[1] Hospitals which had a statistically significant mortality rate more than twice the average in the rest of the English NHS were identified as dangerous. The average mortality rate was 7.4%. Three English hospitals had mortality rates above 14.8% and 30 had rates consistently greater than 7.4%. Units needed to be performing at least 32 operations a year to produce statistically meaningful results, and the units performing the most operations generally got better results. A similar (unpublished) analysis up to March 31, 2007, has again identified three dangerous units.

So why has Bruce Keogh, clinical director of the NHS, said that no unit performing AAA repair is unsafe, despite his own figures showing units with nearly four times the average mortality rate? Why did Lord Darzi, a surgeon himself, not define a statistical safe standard in his tortuous review? And why isn't Barbara Young, *Eye*-reading chair of the new Care Quality Commission, stopping units that can't prove their safety and investigating those where there is proof that they are dangerous? Similar statistical outliers exist for other operations, such as carotid endarterectomy and angioplasty. One lesson from Bristol is that if you collect outcomes, but don't act on the results, you're courting disaster. In the meantime, all patients wanting safe surgery should ask: 'Do you do enough of these procedures to produce statistically meaningful results?' and if so, 'Is your death rate more than

---

[1] Demonstrating safety through in-hospital mortality analysis. *British Journal of Surgery* 2008; 95: 64–71.

double the average elsewhere in the NHS?' Then you have a choice . . .

Danger! GPs at work

11 September 2008

How safe is general practice? No-one really knows, because no-one collects any data. The National Patient Safety Agency has a National Reporting and Learning System (NRLS) for near misses and cock-ups anywhere in the NHS. It's confidential and voluntary, supposedly to encourage participation. Of the 80,000 reports it receives each month, 5% come from community pharmacies and 6% from GPs. Considering 90% of healthcare occurs outside hospitals, it's a piss-poor effort.

There is good evidence from the airline industry, and increasingly from hospitals, that the more errors you report, the less likely you are to harm people. This seems counter-intuitive but organisations that collect, analyse and learn from minor errors are far better at preventing serious ones. Many GP practices have audit meetings behind closed doors, where they discuss complaints, deaths and any bodge-ups that may have been spotted. This is generally done in a supportive, no-blame manner, even when there's clear evidence that someone has made a rudimentary error. And the error is hardly ever reported, least of all by a GP. Most of the NRLS reports from primary care are about vaccination, suggesting they come from nurses.

All clinical staff make mistakes and the error count is rising as medicine becomes more complex. But without a systematic way of picking up and learning from errors, it's likely that the same ones just keep repeating themselves. Recently, I attended a Medicine Safety in Practice conference in Manchester which discussed prescribing errors so serious that they couldn't be hidden. The first concerned a man on long-term warfarin therapy to reduce his risk of a stroke. He also suffered from arthritis. Everyone in the room knew what was going to happen. He was going to take a pain killer that would interact with the warfarin and suffer a catastrophic bleed.

So how did it happen? The patient saw a locum GP on a morning when the computer crashed. The locum didn't know him or ask about his other medications before giving him a prescription for a non-steroidal anti-inflammatory drug (NSAID). His usual pharmacy had a big Christmas queue so he went to an unfamiliar chemist who also didn't check his medications. And his blood test at the warfarin clinic was delayed because of the holidays. He went home, ate some turkey and had a massive stomach bleed.

Most examples showed how heavily GPs rely on their computer to prevent cock-ups, and how simply errors can occur. E.g., a consultant mumbled the name of a drug – triamcinolone – into a tape recorder and it was wrongly transcribed as methotrexate. Not even close. The letter was sent to the GP unchecked. The GP issued a prescription. The pharmacist queried it but was satisfied when the receptionist read the letter back to her. The drug was given as an injection by the practice nurse who didn't realise it was cytotoxic (i.e. able to kill healthy tissue) and got her decimal point in the wrong place, giving ten times the dose. The nurse realised her latter mistake, got the patient into A&E and reported the error. The Primary Care Trust has now banned cytotoxic injections in primary care and offered medicine safety training, which GPs are too busy to attend.

For patients, the best chance of avoiding drug errors is to know what drugs you're taking, what the side effects are and what you can, and can't, take with them. And check the name and dose with whoever is about to inject you. Avoiding misdiagnosis or substandard treatment is harder, but anyone can access Clinical Knowledge Summaries and the Map of Medicine via the NHS Choices website (www.nhs.uk), which give you a good indication of the treatment you should be getting. So there's no excuse for not knowing as much (or even more) than your doctor.

Don't Stop that Pigeon

21 November 2008

'Most entrants were quite apologetic. Connecting for Health hadn't delivered what they wanted so they had to design something themselves that worked.' So said one of the judges at this year's BT e-health Insider Awards when asked why most of the winners were local IT projects and nothing to do with the government's NHS IT programme. Connecting for Health (CfH) has issued a robust defence of itself on its website (www.connectingforhealth.nhs.uk/factsandfiction) but when I read off the '12 most common myths' (e.g. costs are spiralling, the project is plagues with delays, the centralist model is unworkable, the technical architecture is flawed), no-one seemed keen to refute them despite there being a large CfH contingent in the audience.

On the plus side, the NHS Spine and broadband seem to be working OK and PACS, which enables X-rays and scans to be stored electronically and viewed on screens, is working well in many hospitals. And CfH did have one winning entry, a system for assessing what's an emergency and what isn't. It apparently saves 700 inappropriate ambulance journeys a month in the north east alone. Generally, CfH has come unstuck when trying to deliver services at a local level. For example, the NHS Care Records Service (CRS) is supposed to swiftly link patient information from different parts of the NHS electronically, but its roll out at London's Royal Free hospital was a disaster (*Eye* last [give specific date]) Why?

One award judge blamed Richard Granger, the former programme director. 'Granger kicked out anyone who'd previously worked in NHS IT and decided to design an entirely new system from scratch with people who hadn't worked in healthcare. He believed he could control the whole programme from the centre, without learning any of the lessons from the past. But command and control only works with very simple, linear systems. Throw a brick out of the window with a certain force and trajectory, and you can predict where it lands. But healthcare is far more complex, more like a pigeon than a brick. Throw a pigeon and you've no idea where it will land. If you're clever, you get people together locally, decide where you need your pigeon and put down bird seed. If you're Richard Granger, you get the pigeon to land by tying a brick to it.'

In contrast, the Scottish Emergency Care Summary, a simpler equivalent to the English Care Records Service, is up and running well and won an award in the category sponsored by CfH. A Welsh entry also won its category. So what are they doing that the English aren't. As a Welsh IT expert put it: 'Scotland and Wales are smaller communities, with more collaboration and co-operation than the market-obsessed English NHS. They assume that NHS staff are generally trustworthy and have developed 'higher trust' IT systems that are simpler and easier to access, and have managed to gain the consent of patients. Contrast this to England, where no-one can be trusted and the media is paranoid about leakage of confidential data. So you've built hugely complex programmes with military grade security to block the few bad people but which take ages to log onto, navigate around or swap user. At their worst, they stop you practising medicine, rather than enable you to do the job better.'

Granger's parting shot from the IT programme was to boast at how tough his contract negotiations had been, leaving companies such as BT – the award sponsors – with draconian penalties if they don't deliver. But the contracts are so inflexible that delays are inevitable. BT has now had to lay off 10,000 staff partly because it has no successful NHS IT model to sell globally. The NHS may only lose several billion as a result, but the opportunity cost in terms of lives that could have been improved or saved with a working IT system delivered on time, is much greater.

NICE Babies

5 December 2008

Why is the National Institute for Health and Clinical Excellence thriving after 10 years, with annual funding predicted to reach £100 million, when so many other 'new' Labour quangos have bitten the dust? The Modernisation Agency, the NHS University, the Commission for Public and Patient Involvement in Health and the Healthcare Commission have all had their chips, but NICE is bigger than ever, having just landed the contract to host a 'one stop information portal' called NHS Evidence.

At its most basic level, NICE is a firewall between the 'dying mother denied vital cancer drug' stories and government. No politician wants to be trapped in an anguished debate about an individual tragedy, so it's far easier to pass the buck onto NICE. Harder to ascertain is whether NICE delivers value for money. It has now produced so much guidance that it's in danger of devoting all of its resources to updating what it already has, rather than assess new treatments. And is there any evidence that its guidance actually get used on the frontline to improve care for patients?

I have been to the last three NICE conferences and the highlight is always the competition for those who've put the evidence into action. This year's winner was an obstetric team from North Bristol NHS Trust, who wanted to reduce brain damage to babies during birth. This is still a huge problem. The seventh Confidential Enquiry into Stillbirth and Disability in Infancy found much the same as the previous six; in 75% of cases there was evidence of poor care, most frequently a failure to interpret electronic foetal monitoring (EFM).

NICE concluded in 2001, that delays in recognising and acting on the signs of suspected foetal distress could lead to prolonged resuscitation at birth, brain damage due to a lack of oxygen and increased risk of cerebral palsy. This is not just a human tragedy. Claims for cerebral palsy arising from negligent obstetric care cost the NHS more than claims for all other specialties put together.

NICE recommended that all maternity staff should receive annual training in EFM, and that outcome measures of oxygen starvation, such as 5-minute APGAR scores (which assess the baby's vital signs) should be monitored. The North Bristol team managed to get everyone to turn up to training, from the most junior midwife to the most senior obstetrician, and devised a simple sticker for the notes to ensure all members of staff recorded the EFM in a standardised way, even if they were knackered and trying to look after more than one labouring woman at the same time.

The sticker makes it easy to spot when the EFM trace is normal, suspicious or pathological, and when to call for urgent senior support. As a result, problems are spotted earlier, low APGAR scores have halved and the number of babies showing signs of brain damage due to lack of oxygen has fallen by nearly two thirds. The annual training course costs less than £20 per member of staff, easily offset by the savings in litigation.

The NHS has a fine record of innovation and improvement, but it usually doesn't spread across the board. The NICE website has a 'shared learning database' but to use it, NHS staff need time to focus on the evidence of what works, rather than running around trying to implement un-evidence based reform. If the Darzi review is true to its word, puts evidence at the heart of healthcare and backs it up with adequate training, it might actually improve care. And it could even save money.

More Top-Ups

29 December 2008

Should top up prescriptions be extended beyond cancer drugs? The debate following the report by cancer tsar Mike Richards – *Improving Access to Medicines for NHS Patients* – concentrated on what are touchingly known as 'end of life medicines' (i.e. drugs that cost thousands of pounds in return for a few extra months of breathing). But there are plenty more mundane drugs that the NHS is refusing to fund and that patients should at least be offered the chance to buy – if appropriate – for the lowest possible price. This already happens with prescriptions for malaria prevention and erectile dysfunction, where patients have their consultation as part of the NHS and just have to pay for the cost of the drugs privately. In theory, GPs can issue private prescriptions for any licensed drug, even if NICE has given it the thumbs down, but in practice, this rarely happens.

When NICE restricts the use of a drug on the NHS, the issue is not that it doesn't work at all, but that it doesn't work well enough, in their judgement, to justify the cost. So use is either not recommended or strictly limited. A further complication is that although NICE's remit supposedly extends to public health, for some bizarre reason it doesn't evaluate vaccines or screening programmes. Vaccination recommendations come from the Joint Committee on Vaccination and Immunisation (JCVI), and although flu vaccination is one of the best ways of avoiding flu (along with not letting someone with flu sneeze, cough or wipe their snot on you), the JCVI only sanctions free jabs for those at highest risk of death from flu (i.e. over 65 or with certain chronic diseases). Flu vaccines are often in limited supply but this year we have plenty that have not been used and, given the largest outbreak for 8 years, the misery caused by influenza and the economic cost of time off work, it would seem sensible to offer the surplus as an NHS top-up to those under 65 who want to protect themselves.

If you do get flu, there are anti-viral drugs that can prevent the virus from replicating, reduce the duration of symptoms and likelihood of complications, and get you back to work more quickly. The effects are significant, though not huge, but as a course of treatment typically costs £20, NICE decided back in 2003 that NHS treatment should again be restricted to high-risk groups only. However, many healthy people who have suffered flu would happily pay £20 for the chance of the illness being curtailed. However, getting a private prescription is extremely difficult because the drugs are only effective if taken in the first few days of the illness, and the NHS actively discourages anyone with flu from seeing a doctor unless they're moribund. (Stay at home, avoid all physical contact and wipe your nose on your elbow, not your hand are the three top tips this year from flu experts). So virtually no-one gets anti-viral drugs, not even those who NICE says should have them. Allowing pharmacists to diagnose flu and dispense anti-viral drugs – both privately and on the NHS – might be a solution.

Back in vaccine-land, the JCVI chose Cervarix for the NHS cervical cancer vaccine programme, which only protects against cervical cancer and not against genital and laryngeal warts. The JCVI used an arbitrary points system to reach its decision which seems to bear very little resemblance to the NICE evaluation process, and has repeatedly refused to reveal the price it's paying for the vaccine. Information about an alternative vaccine (Gardasil) with broader disease coverage was completely absent from the NHS Choices (sic) website until the *Eye* pointed it out, and now merits just a sentence. So while those in the know (i.e. doctors) are covertly paying privately for their daughters to have Gardasil, most people are getting no choice at all. The Common's Health Committee is currently inquiring into top-ups. They will hopefully conclude that patients should be given accurate and information about all licensed drugs, and then be given the chance to top up, if clinically indicated. The NHS may not be able to afford everything, but its absurd to deny choice to those patients who can pay a bit more for drugs but can't afford a private GP, even if such a thing existed.

Checking up on Surgery

16 January 2009
Will the much-trumpeted WHO surgical safety checklist reduce cock-ups in the NHS? The research results are certainly promising. In eight pilot sites around the world, use of the checklist cut death rates following surgery from 1.5% to 0.8% and complication rates from 11% to 7%. The absolute risk of surgery is relatively low but given that surgery is now more common than childbirth, with 234 million operations globally a year, introduction of the checklist has the potential to save millions of lives. But only if it's implemented properly.

The UK pilot site for the study was Lord Darzi's hunting ground – St Mary's hospital, Paddington – but only two operating theatres were enrolled, not including the one where a gynaecology patient had her gall bladder erroneously removed. This 'wrong patient, wrong site, wrong organ' calamity will doubtless give Darzi the leverage to implement the checklist in his own trust, but what about the rest of the NHS?

The strategy of the National Patient Safety Agency (NPSA)

is to issue an alert requiring anyone performing surgery in the NHS to use it by February 2010. All organisations (NHS and private) will have to submit to an audit to prove compliance, and any stragglers will receive a visit from the new Care Quality Commission. The UK is the first to attempt across-the-board implementation (at least in England and Wales), but the NPSA has to inspire surgical teams to do use the checklist properly. The department of health's previous edict that all ward staff should be bare below the elbows makes common sense (you can't wash thoroughly with coughs in the way) but met with widespread resistance because there is no evidence yet that it reduces the spread of infection. The checklist seems to have a firmer evidence-base, but why should a banal list of blindingly obvious basic safety checks make such a difference? Medicine is now so complex and time-pressured, with many competing demands, that the human brain can't process it safely without the help of aide memoirs. One patient a day is listed for the wrong operation in the NHS and one patient a month gets wrong-site surgery. Last year's Chief Medical Officer's (CMO) report highlighted fourteen patients who'd had holes drilled in the wrong side of their head. Patients suffer and die, and hugely complex and costly surgery is ruined, because antibiotics or clot-preventing drugs aren't given in time.

The checklist may work not just because it forces someone to tick a box but because each item has to be read out loud and agreed by every member of the surgical team, who have all introduced themselves by name and explained their role. Some NHS staff might find this all a bit embarrassing and un-British, and it may just be that the checklist was effective because of the Hawthorne effect: everyone knew they were being observed so they upped their game. In the unobserved NHS, the temptation may just be to take the piss out of it. However, the most telling feedback came from 229 surgeons involved in the study. 80% felt it had improved safety and reduced errors, and 92.6%

would want the checklist to be used if they were having an operation. So why wait until February 2010? If you're having an operation – NHS or private – don't sign the consent form until you have written assurance that the checklist is being used. Better still, download it, take it in with you and stick it to your chest. http://www.npsa.nhs.uk/nrls/alerts-and-directives/alerts/safer-surgery-alert/.

A Surgeon Rants ...

24 February 2009

Substandard surgery in Independent Sector Treatment Centres (ISTCs) has been evident for ages but the Royal College of Surgeons (RCS) was shit-scared to rock the boat, for fear of its power being given to the Postgraduate Medical Education and Training Board (PMETB). This has happened anyway, and the RCS is now of largely historical interest, posing around pompously but with zero influence.

The Darzi report claims to be about quality but the ISTCs were purely about numbers. All sorts of surgeons were brought in who would not have passed even slight evaluation against the old standards, but due to European law are allowed to work in the UK. I have just interviewed a young Polish surgeon. He has a European Certificate of Surgical Training (CST) and can come here and work as a specialist, even though he has done the stunning total of 7 laprascopic cholecystectomies (keyhole gall bladder removals).

Meanwhile, we have hundreds of good surgeons

from India, Pakistan and Egypt who learned surgery from British textbooks and then came here and worked for years in our system. As non-Europeans, they were made to jump through ludicrous hoops to become cannon fodder sub-consultant doctors and many have now been sent home. Yet their expertise is way ahead of the new crop of slightly trained UK surgeons we are about to let loose, and of most trainees from Europe.

Because of the hours' restrictions of the European Working Time Directive, surgical trainees are no longer around to learn how to operate on rare and unusual cases, and to deal with the complications. The government and our medical 'leaders' are presiding over a serious decline in surgical standards which will have effects much more widespread than the Bristol affair.

Andrew McIrvine

Complimentary, for Once ...

29 February 2009

A year-long pilot scheme in Northern Ireland found impressive health benefits for patients offered complementary therapies, so why were its findings not released for over a year? 713 patients with physical and/or mental health conditions were referred to various therapies via nine GP practices in Belfast and Londonderry. Patients assessed their own health pre- and post-therapy. After treatment, 80% of patients reported an improvement in their symptoms, 64% took less time off work and 55% reduced their use of painkillers.

The trial wasn't randomised or controlled, so we don't know

how the patients would have fared if given the standard treatment of grumpy nihilism and Ibuprofen. But the fact that so many GPs were won over by the study (99% said they would refer patients to the scheme in future and in 98% said they would recommend the service to other GPs), suggests there might be something in it. The fact that the Northern Ireland health board hasn't released the results in a big fanfare suggests they don't have the money to extend the service. Judge for yourself at: http://www.dhsspsni.gov.uk/final_report_from_ smr_ on_the_cam_pilot_project_-_may_2008.pdf

Not so complimentary . . .

13 March 2009

The Northern Irish survey that found an overwhelmingly positive response to the use of complementary and alternative medicine (CAM) in general practice provoked a mixed response from *Eye* readers. Joseph O'Connor was unimpressed: 'Without a control group or any randomisation, the trial tells us diddly squat. What CAM treatments have in common is an opportunity for the patient to simply talk to someone and to feel that something is being done about their problem; prime opportunity for the placebo effect to kick in and something which GPs cannot currently do as a result of their heavy workloads.

'The website of Get Well UK, which ran the project, states that some of the benefits of CAM are the relationship with the practitioner, and the opportunity for that person to take a detailed case history. Rather than referring patients to unproven therapies from those with little medical training, we should increase the number of GPs, so that appointments do not need to be crammed into narrow windows and patients can feel as if they are more than walking illnesses to their doctors.'

David Colquhoun, a pipe-smoking professor of pharmacology at University College, London was even more scathing: 'It's not that I'm against the human side of medicine, just that I want it done honestly. To give people sugar pills accompanied by a bunch of lies is condescending, disempowering and dishonest. I can well understand that there are a lot of people whom GPs would like to get off their backs (not least in Northern Ireland it seems) but there must be an honest way to do it. Any practice made up of GPs with half-decent critical faculties would probably never have got mixed up with a study that was so obviously incapable of telling you anything useful or new.'

CAM therapies exist because people find them helpful, irrespective of whether their treatment is more than placebo. Marjorie Titchen is 91 years old and still runs a small hotel in Bournemouth. She has worked and paid tax for 75 years and is unimpressed that Bournemouth and Poole Teaching Primary Care Trust won't fund homeopathy for her osteoarthritis even though they have done in the past and she's found it to be by far the most effective treatment she's had (and much less likely to burn a hole in her stomach than Ibuprofen).

The PCT has withdrawn treatment because 'there is no scientific evidence to support it.' But there's plenty of evidence to support the use of placebos and good communication skills, and there's no guarantee that Mrs Titchen would get either from a random succession of stressed GPs. Having found something that works for her, she wants to stick to it.

As the money dries up in the NHS, it's likely that complementary therapies will be squeezed out along with care of the elderly. The best way for CAM to get NHS funding is to produce conclusive trial evidence, and the NHS now has a vast GP research database that can be used for randomised observational studies of 'real life' patients, rather than the more artificial environment of controlled trials.[1] The database is ideally suited to CAM research and overseen by Dr John Parkinson (BSc, PhD), a pharmacoepidemiologist who also trained in traditional Chinese medicine. All that's needed is the funding. Perhaps Prince Charles could donate the profits from his Duchy Herbals' artichoke and dandelion detox tincture (£10 for 50ml)

The Mid Staffs Scandal – Not Learning From Bristol

27 March 2009

'The culture of the future must be a culture of safety and of quality; a culture of openness and accountability: a culture of public service ... Safety requires constant vigilance ... The government must organise good, comprehensive and independent systems to mange to regulate the quality of healthcare ... Chief executives are legally responsible for monitoring and improving the quality of healthcare, and must be supported and enabled to carry out this duty ... At trust board level, an executive should be responsible for putting into action the trust's strategy and policy on safety and a non-executive director should provide leadership to promote a culture of safety. And when things go wrong, patients are entitled to receive an acknowledgement, an explanation and an apology.'

So concluded the Bristol Royal Infirmary Inquiry in July 2001. Of its 198 recommendations, very few seem to have been implemented at Mid Staffordshire Foundation Trust, where as many as 1,200 patients may have died due to poor emergency

---

[1] http://www.gprd.com/home/

treatment. Health secretary Alan Johnson has ordered an inquiry going back to 2002, when the problems seem to have started. So why did it take the Healthcare Commission (HC) until 2009 to publicise such 'shockingly poor care?'

In 1992, when the *Eye* exposed the Bristol scandal, the Conservative government awarded the Bristol Royal Infirmary its Charter Mark for Excellence, despite the appalling mortality rates for child heart surgery. Likewise, Mid Staffs reached the pinnacle of new Labour achievement – foundation trust status – despite the corporate manslaughter of hundreds of patients. Labour has played lip service to the Bristol Inquiry, creating an NHS obsessed with performance (hitting financial and activity targets). So a hospital with lots of ticked boxes and a sky-high death rate can gain huge financial rewards and independence from Whitehall.

The regulatory system that was supposed to come in post-Bristol has clearly failed. David Nicholson, now chief executive of the NHS, held senior management positions in the West Midlands between 2001 and 2006, and was succeeded by Cynthia Bowyer until 2008, when she became chief executive of the latest health watchdog (the Care Quality Commission). Yet neither seem to have a clue what was going on under their noses in Mid Staffs.

Bower claims she could have acted sooner if the HC (which the CQC is replacing) had shared its data. The HC claims that West Midlands Strategic Health Authority was 'difficult to engage.' A separate regulatory body, Monitor, was set up to vet and monitor foundation trusts. It clearly hasn't got a clue about quality either and has had a very frosty and competitive relationship with the HC. Since 2003, the HC has been chaired by Ian Kennedy as his reward for chairing the Bristol Inquiry. The HC took over from the Commission for Health Improvement (CHI), which awarded Mid Staffs a top 'three star' rating in 2002–03. But according to the Health Service

Journal, former Mid Staffs non-executive director David Denny was unimpressed. 'The board was somewhat puzzled. We didn't believe the standards were as high as they needed to be.'

So why wasn't something done? Ultimate responsibility lies with the leadership in the hospital. In May 2007, Wrightington, Wigan and Leigh NHS trust was told that its death rates were one of the highest in the NHS (and not far short of Mid Staffs). But instead of challenging and denying the data, the chief executive Andrew Foster accepted it, got the board and clinical staff behind him and did something about it, getting all the staff to focus on quality and safety. As a result, mortality rates have dropped by 15%, saving 200 lives a year.

But perhaps the most important lesson from Bristol is that anyone on the frontline – staff, patient or relative – needs to be encouraged to speak up and have their concerns acted on. For every scandal in the NHS, the whistle has been blown long before the establishment has acted. The Stafford campaign group Cure the NHS knew perfectly well how appalling the care was because their relatives were on the receiving end. The most enlightened NHS trusts encourage patients and relatives to feedback and use bedside software that allows instant monitoring of complaints (poor hygiene, wrong tablets, no food, drinking from vases). As the visionary Bristol anaesthetist Steve Bolsin observed: 'If you want to prevent future disasters, you must never lose sight of the patient.'

Note: MD has signed the petition for an independent inquiry into the Mid Staffs scandal (as opposed to a New Labour fudge) at: www.patients-association.com

More Staffing Problems

8 April 2009

A key question for the investigation into the appalling standards of emergency care at Mid Staffordshire hospital is: 'Why did no member of staff blow the whistle sooner?' In a 2006 Healthcare Commission survey, only 27% of the Mid Staffs staff said they would be happy to be treated in their own hospital, a powerful indication that standards were unacceptable. And after Bristol, the General Medical Council deemed that doctors had a duty to speak up when the service becomes so unsafe that patients are being harmed.

However, the experience of Dr Rita Pal in nearby North Staffs suggests that whistle-blowing in the NHS remains a thankless task. Dr Pal identified serious shortcomings in the nursing and medical care of patients on Ward 87 of City General Hospital, Stoke on Trent, when she started working there in August 1998. These included a lack of basic equipment such as drip sets, a lack of adequate support and supervision for junior doctors, a gross shortage of staff and repeated 'do not resuscitate' notices. As a result, patient care was often poor, with a lack of baseline observations and routine blood tests, and there appeared to be an unacceptably high mortality rate.

In November 1998, Dr Pal articulated these concerns to senior nursing and medical staff, and put them in writing. As a result, she was bullied and victimised. She was wrongly accused of causing a needle-stick injury and inserting the wrong date on a drug sheet, and she found out that her previous consultant had been contacted to ascertain whether she was 'capable of doing the job' (i.e. flying by the seat of her pants with inadequate support and resources, surrounded by hostile nursing staff and patients dying unnecessarily). She requested leave because she (quite reasonably) felt unable to care for patients in this environment.

Subsequent investigation found that Dr Pal's allegations had been spot on. A review in May 1999 by Mrs T Fenech from the Infectious Diseases Unit found 'serious deficiencies in nursing practice' and that 'the level of care demonstrated for some patients on the ward at the time of my audit was nothing short of negligent.' In 2001, an internal report concluded that the directorate failed to take appropriate action when the allegations were made by Dr Pal and that patients had suffered from poor standards of care. And in March 2002, the Commission for Health Improvement still found 'serious deficiencies' particularly with 'the level of supervision, work-load and work patterns of junior doctors working within medicine.'

So not only were Dr Pal's initial allegations accurate, but four years later very little had been done to address them. Dr Pal took her concerns to the General Medical Council and – eleven years after first raising concerns – is still embroiled in a fight to ascertain the true extent of the harm done to patients on Ward 87. A mature and safety-conscious NHS would have thanked her for raising concerns to help improve patient care, and acted on them. Instead, she has been bullied, falsely accused of malpractice and repeatedly denied access to key documents to help support her case.

Last week, Sir Ian Kennedy, retiring chair of the Healthcare Commission, spoke of the bullying culture in the NHS that still 'permeates the delivery of care.' Those who are brave enough to speak up about deficiencies in care are being pilloried and silenced. In such an environment, patient safety can never flourish. Dr Pal has lobbied (via her MP Andrew Mitchell) for the Commons Health Select Committee to investigate the problems faced by whistle-blowers in the NHS. She has also started a support network for whistle-blowers and can be contacted at: dr.ritapal@googlemail.com

Struck Off and Die

23 April 2009

Why was whistle-blowing nurse Margaret Haywood struck off by the Nursing and Midwifery Council (NMC)? Haywood admitted to breaching patient confidentiality by secretly filming and passing on information about elderly patients at Brighton and Sussex NHS Hospital trust to the *Panorama* team. But given the appalling standards of care she exposed, she could legitimately claim this was in the public interest. Patients, relatives and staff members had been complaining about lack of basic nursing on Peel and Stewart wards since the Summer of 2004, with little effect, and it took the 'undercover nurse' documentary to force the trust to act and protect future patients from harm.

No patient or relative complained about Haywood's actions, and the BBC sought the consent of every patient who made the final edit (or their next of kin). Haywood realized from the outset that in passing the tapes onto journalists she was in breach of her duty of care but was convinced (probably rightly) that without such a graphic exposure of the failings, nothing was likely to be done. Breaches of confidentiality are permissible by the NMC (and the Public Interest Disclosure Act) in extreme circumstances, such as when patients are suffering significant harm, and although this was undoubtedly the case, Hayward's undoing was the fact that this information was not used urgently to protect the patients she filmed. Filming took place between November 3, 2004 and May 5, 2005, but the programme didn't air until July 20 and very few of the patients featured (some of whom were terminally ill) benefited from their confidentiality being breached.

Haywood was also unable to prove that the she might have achieved a similar effect by 'going through the correct channels' but countless NHS whistle-blowers would testify to the futility of this route. It was the trust that reported her to the NMC and threw in an absurd allegation that she had failed to assist when a patient had a grand mal convulsion. This was found to be groundless by the NMC but the smearing of whistle-blowers is a depressingly common tactic used to discredit them, and her chances of being listened to as a bank nurse raising concerns internally were close to zero.

Haywood's actions helped to improve nursing care for patients at the trust, and she has the support of many patients and relatives, fellow nurses and even the Royal College of Nursing. In reporting her, the trust may have reduced, or possibly increased, its chances of falling prey to covert filming in future, and has attracted a lot of bad press. How do you explain that a nurse who exposes bad practice is struck off, and yet those who dish it out or oversee it remain in employment?

It is the NMC that comes out of it looking most foolish. The finding of breach of confidentiality was not unexpected, but at 58, and with the stress of a ludicrously protracted investigation that concluded nearly four years after the event, Haywood has no desire to participate in future filming. Besides, her cover is blown. Most nurses believe that her bravery has enhanced, rather than harmed, the reputation of nursing. Her nursing record is good and she is not a risk to patients. The wise option would have been to caution her but, in striking her off, the NMC has merely demonstrated how out of touch it is with the nurses it seeks to regulate and the public it claims to serve. Indeed, the backlash has been so strong, that the NMC has retreated even further into its self-protective shell. As its website warns: 'abusive or threatening emails and telephone calls to NMC staff will be noted and may be passed to the relevant authorities for further action.' Meanwhile, NHS staff will feel even less inclined to speak up about dangerous and substandard care.

The 48-Hour Week

7 May 2009

John Black, President of the Royal College of Surgeons, strayed off-message at this month's Patient Safety Congress in Birmingham: 'Patient choice doesn't work. The one area where quality and safety have improved year on year is the one area where patients don't currently have any choice. Cancer care.' His observation is backed up by an analysis by the Picker Institution and the *Health Service Journal* which found that, a year after patients were given free choice to go wherever they wanted, most still go to their local hospital and there is no evidence yet that choice is driving up standards.

Black was also dismissive of the current obsession with data protection and confidentiality: 'Some hospitals won't allow doctors to e-mail scans and X-rays to each other. On wards, vital information like temperature charts and blood pressure readings are locked away so no-one can look at them. And often patient names aren't even displayed above the bed, which makes life very confusing for the cardiac arrest team.'

But Black reserved particular ire, and several bright yellow slides with red lettering, for the European Working Time Directive (EWTD), which means that junior doctors are not allowed to average more than 48 hours a week from August 1. 'It was designed for Spanish lorry drivers and is making the NHS far less safe, with dangerously thin layers of medical cover, poor training and multiple handovers.' Black trained in an era when junior doctors might be on duty for over 120 hours a week (admittedly not always working), and is clearly outraged by anyone doing so little: 'Surgeons can't be safely trained for the future and provide a safe level of cover across the NHS with a 48-hour week.'

Not everyone agrees. There is good evidence that the fatigue of long hours and sleep deprivation affects a doctor's performance and the NHS has had 11 years to prepare for the 48-hour legal limit. Some hospitals, such as Homerton in East London, hit the target over a year ago, but it required a change in consultants hours from 9 a.m.–5 p.m. to 8 a.m.–10 p.m. (they get paid for it), putting them in charge of emergency admissions and making space for training. But above all, you need sufficient junior staff to work the day or night shift system.

This is where the EWTD seems to be falling apart in parts of the NHS. Last year's cock-up over junior doctors' job applications left a big dent in the hospital workforce as many left for Australia and New Zealand, or jumped ship to general practice. And the sending home of Asian doctors combined with the falling pound, which has made the NHS less attractive to European trainees, has left gaping holes in many shift rotas. Across the country, some specialties are operating with less than half the required number of junior staff, with knackered consultants desperately having to backfill the shifts. Or not. When I qualified in 1987, it was not uncommon for a single junior doctor to be left alone to cover dozens of patients across many wards at night. Fast forward 22 years to the Mid Stafford fiasco, and a single, very junior surgeon was left alone to look after every surgical patient in the hospital at night.

Safe staffing levels are the key to patient safety, and the EWTD was supposed to be introduced alongside a consultant-led service where supervision was always available and training opportunities were maximised. Some hospitals have had the foresight to implement this. Those that haven't have no chance of hitting the 48-hour target in two months time but will have to look as if they are. Without sufficient staff, medical cover will go from dangerously thin to non-existent in parts. For once, the Royal College of Surgeons may have a point.

Impatient Feedback

10 May 2009

Dear MD,

Sorry, but John Black does NOT have a point about patient choice. Giving us choice but denying us the information we'd need in order to use that choice is no more than a deliberate attempt to undermine the principle of choice, and both you and he must know that quite well.

I'm sick to the back teeth of hearing fatuous arguments like this. I have heard a twerp from Stafford hospital saying recently that we locals must still trust the hospital as some of us are still going there. What else are we expected to do? Cancel appointments with consultants we've been waiting months for and start all over again at another hospital with a consultant taken out of a hat because our GP only knows the local consultants? Cancel surgery we've been waiting months for and start again elsewhere from the beginning? In any case, *some* wards are very good there. But which ones, and how do we find out, except by personal experience of friends and family? There isn't always someone you know who has the same illness you do.

We peasants will only be able to 'choose' when we are also given true and full information about which hospitals are crap, which wards are filthy, which places are staffed with bone idle nurses and which surgeons couldn't find their arse with both hands. And who/what is blocking us finding out?

At present, even the NHS itself doesn't know, and it is happy to believe any old crap hospitals choose to tell it, even when patients have been (literally) going blue in the face complaining.

I have recently been treated by an excellent surgeon (who, incidentally, I would love to recommend to other patients for his kindness, skill and high professional standards, but of course there is no way I can do that) but in a completely crap hospital. I *chose* to go there on the basis of my experience years ago, when it was a good hospital. I could not have found out about the current atrocious nursing standards there by any other means. Its last inspection was years ago, it isn't due for another for years, and the only information online I could find was a report on the Healthcare Commission site that gave it full marks in all respects. I subsequently found that this was not a proper inspection report, but had been compiled simply from the hospital's own written submissions, and was not a result of an inspection by an impartial authority. My experience was so totally different from the report I thought I'd read the wrong page at first. NHS patients may also be 'choosing' to go there on the basis of inadequate information like this.

As far as the NHS goes, here in Stafford, we know to our cost that relying on a hospital's report of its performance is about as sensible as believing that there are fairies at the bottom of the garden. We have known that A&E here is crap for a long time, but no-one listened, (and no doctors seem to have tried to do anything about it) and where the hell are we supposed to go when we are in a RTA or have a heart attack anyway? What choice do we have then? For non-emergency work, even my GP couldn't recommend anyone outside the local hospital because she only knows the surgeons who work there. So how do I choose if I want to go elsewhere when even my GP hasn't access to enough information to help me choose? Where do I go to to find out who's an idiot and who is at least a safe choice?

It's okay for you doctors – you can ask around your colleagues and they'll tell you the truth on the quiet about the consultants/hospitals/GPs they know – but what about us?

Until no reports are made public that are not the result of thorough and independent inspections we'll be totally in the dark, so how the hell can we choose?

Without details of the success rates of the specific surgeon we will see, for the surgery we are having, how can we choose? Without getting access to all complaints on a by-hospital, by-ward, and by-surgeon basis, how can we choose?

The present system is like telling us we can have the gold ingot over *there*, but chaining us to the the tree over *here*. And then saying, 'look, you haven't picked up the ingot . . . you obviously never really wanted it, we knew you didn't but you wouldn't listen to us.'

And so we have to guess where to go. Guess wrong on this one, and you're dead. Russian roulette, in fact. Some choice.

Yours, getting increasingly cheesed off,
Alison Wilson

And on a Brighter Note ...

19 May 2009

Dear Phil

You have already given us more positive coverage than I have ever seen in *Private Eye* but I thought you might still be interested to see how things ended up so I attach our first ever Quality Account.

The headlines are that year on year, our Hospital Standardised Mortality Rate went down from 125.7 (07–08) to 92.8 (08–09) and year on year actual deaths went down from 1561 (07–08) to 1347 (08–09). I don't suppose that we will manage to abolish death altogether but the downward trend continues and there were just 75 deaths in Month 1 (April 2009) compared to 126 in the same month last year.

In the interests of balance I would confess that we had a poor A&E performance, missed our MRSA target by one and failed to achieve our financial surplus target. I think we could argue though that death rates are more important than government targets.

Best wishes

Andrew Foster

Chief Executive

Wrightington, Wigan & Leigh NHS Foundation Trust

ANDY BURNHAM
June 2009–

Health Secretary was one of the deckchairs to be filled in Gordon Brown's hasty reshuffle. A thankless job at the best of times, it's likely to get a whole lot harder as the money dries up and the NHS has to make cuts to pay off the public debt. Denham turned it down, Balls only has eyes for the Treasury, Darling wasn't budging and Flint was too female (allegedly). So come in Andy Burnham, the first health secretary to be younger than me (by some eight years).

Little Boy Burnham is an Indie-loving Everton fan, but he isn't entirely green. He's been on the Commons Health Select Committee and held the gloriously Stalinesque office of Minister of State for Delivery and Reform at the Department of Health, before he jumped ship to culture and a Boris Johnson bonding-session with Liverpool fans. His expenses were some of the first to be blown by the *Telegraph*, including a letter to the Fees Office begging for a £16,000 decorating bill to be paid: 'otherwise I might be in line for divorce!' And a large part of a windfall from his landlord was then effectively added to his second home allowance (all within the rules, apparently). On a brighter note, he had a £19.99 claim for an Ikea bathrobe harshly rejected. Ideal for hiding in the bathroom when the decorators pop round with the bill.

Whether he can get to grips with the complex NHS finances in the fag end of Labour remains to be seen. As a Blairite, he may want to safeguard the legacy of his reforms but he needn't worry too much. If you cut up the current Labour and Tory health plans (which is quite therapeutic in itself) and mix them up, it's very hard to tell them apart. The English NHS, at least, appears stuck with a dysfunctional market that's fast running out of money. The ideological fault line between those who believe in competition as the best way to provide a health service, and those wedded to co-operation, is now so deep that it appears unbridgeable. The Department of Health is trying to come up with a third way – 'co-opetition'– but we've had our fill of 'new' Labour bullshit. Labour still argues fervently that patients want choice, and I tend to agree. But only if the choice is based on meaningful and useful information. After twelve years of Labour, we still don't have accurate, comparative outcome data or defined safety standards to protect patients. Not all this is Labour's fault – quality and safety need to be grown from the bottom up, and it's up to NHS staff to lead the charge. But politicians have to embrace this focus on quality and safety, not bury it under the guff of needless reform and secretive competition. Andrew Lansley take note.

PRIVATE EYE
Pathological Sickness

10 June 2009

On June 1, 2007 a letter was sent to Dr Martin Morse, Medical Director of North Bristol Trust (NBT), detailing eleven alleged serious diagnostic errors made by histopathologists at the Bristol Royal Infirmary (BRI), resulting in significant patient harm. These cases came to light when slides and samples were subsequently reviewed at NBT.

According to the allegations, one woman (now deceased) was told her breast biopsy was benign but later presented with metastatic cancer, and patients with malignant lymphoma, melanoma (twice) and vulval carcinoma were also initially told they did not have cancer. Conversely, two other patients allegedly had treatment for cancer when review of their biopsies found no evidence of it.

Documented errors appeared most likely in patients with rare lung disease. Again, patients have allegedly been told they have cancer when they don't and vice versa. Another was allegedly told he had tuberculosis when subsequent review found that he didn't.

Interpreting tissue slides is stressful and complex, and some mistakes inevitably happen. The Royal College of Pathologists (RCPath) states that when discrepancies in reporting occur, prompt independent review is required but some of these errors date back to 2000, and when the college was invited to do such a review, it apparently declined.

Bristol is blessed with some fine pathologists, including respiratory specialists based at NBT, and if they worked in teams, accepted the same quality control and shared difficult diagnoses, then doubtless some harm to patients could have been prevented or reduced.

Alas, the long-standing rivalry and competition between Bristol hospitals has prevented this from happening. Until July 2008, NBT pathologists claim they were unable to access the slides for their patients who were treated at the BRI, though this has now been resolved. However, slides from other patients who might benefit from the specialist service at NBT are still not being shared. Dr Morse has raised concerns with the Medical Director of University Hospitals Bristol (UHB), Dr Jonathan Sheffield but – two years after the whistle was blown – an independent external review has not happened. Four additional cases of apparent lung misdiagnosis have now been documented, but Dr Sheffield has stated that there is 'no evidence to confirm a significant error rate' in the service.

As well as the RCPath, these concerns have been brought to the attention of the chief executives of both trusts, the medical director of the strategic health authority, the medical director of the Avon Somerset and Wiltshire Cancer Services and the National Clinical Assessment Authority, thus far without satisfactory investigation or resolution.

It seems extraordinary, given what happened previously in Bristol, that UHB staff would not accept they might have a problem in their pathology department and act quickly to get an outside assessment. An urgent external review and the assimilation of pathology services across Bristol into a network that encourages scrutiny and shared expertise is now vital for patient safety. Dr Sheffield has been sent a detailed summary of the alleged misdiagnoses and I have asked the RCPath and the Care Quality Commission to investigate.

Labour's Pains

24 June 2009

New health secretary Andy Burnham does a fine line in cheesy tributes, describing his predecessor Alan Johnson as 'the postman who delivered for the NHS.' But Johnson got out just in time, leaving Burnham (39, Capricorn) to pick up a number of suspicious packages: The swine flu pandemic, a predicted Summer heat-wave, a staffing crisis caused by the 48-hour week for junior doctors and a projected five-year shortfall in NHS funding of £20 billion. Alas, his maiden speech at the NHS Confederation conference did little to inspire confidence: "Can we do more to get through the challenge and to the next level, going from good to world-class?"

He also promised to "unlock the 1.4 million people working in the NHS" and "create a truly people-centred NHS – which genuinely empowers patients and carers as experts potentially backed with control over funds, moving on heath promotion and physical activity, helping people to lead full happy lives, working with public sector partners to wrap care around patients and to place quality at heart of everything". Burnham is clearly au fait with new Labour bullshit, but can he stop the NHS going tits up in the recession?

The NHS has undoubtedly got better over the last decade, but there are still huge variations in the quality of care, and plenty of commercial secrecy and petty rivalry disguising poor practice and waste. Lord Darzi has been frantically encouraging doctors to get more involved in management, and it certainly makes sense for a clinical service to be run by clinicians. But the English NHS is stuck with a market which hasn't delivered a good enough service because nobody knows how to spend £100 billion a year without wasting half of it.

The solution was supposed to be word class commissioning (WCC), a phrase dreamt up by Mark Britnell, the self-styled NHS director general for commissioning and system management. Britnell also came up with the FESC framework to encourage the private sector to take control of the purse strings.

Britnell was the golden boy of the department of health, voted third most influential person in the NHS by the Health Service Journal, a chief executive in waiting. Until he jumped ship this month to join KMPG, one of the companies involved in FESC. The revolving door from NHS policy maker to the private health provider is hardly new (Simon Stevens, Alan Milburn, Patricia Hewitt, Lord Warner, Baroness Jay etc) but for Britnell to time his escape as Burnham arrives does not bode well for the NHS or for Burnham.

Has Bristol learned from Bristol?

7 July 2009

How much has the safety culture at University Hospitals Bristol (UHB) changed since the public inquiry into cardiac surgery? On the plus side, when the *Eye* broke the heart scandal in 1992, it took seven years to announce an external inquiry. When allegations of serious histopathology errors were published last month, it took seven days. There's even a web page dedicated to the histopathology review. (www.uhbristol.nhs.uk/histopathology-review-june-2009)

But there's still plenty of 'old' Bristol. Too much power concentrated in too few hands, very serious allegations not shared with the trust board, arrogance and bullying, a shortage of specialist staff, an ineffectual royal college and brave consultants who raised concerns but were not taken seriously. And once again, many doctors, managers and establishment figures have been well aware of the problems for some years, but virtually no patients.

The UHB website says the review was ordered after '15 potential cases of histopathology misdiagnosis' were published in 'the satirical magazine, *Private Eye*.' But the trust knows that there are far more than 15 alleged errors dating back from 2000. These are a sample of the errors collated by a single consultant where significant harm to patients had occurred. There are other examples where harm was fortuitously averted. Other consultants have also raised concerns specifically in four areas (respiratory, breast, skin and gynaecology), some as far back as 2004.

Last year, UHB medical director Jonathan Sheffield and chief executive Graham Rich were also informed of diagnostic errors and omissions in gynaecology reporting picked up by a specialist pathologist over a 2-year-period with 'serious implications for patient safety.' An external expert confirmed the more serious errors.

Dr Sheffield, himself a histopathologist, has frequently met and exchanged correspondence, with those raising concerns but to no satisfactory resolution. In July 2008, the minutes of the Medical Advisory Committee at neighbouring North Bristol Trust (NBT), state that there 'continued to be serious cases of respiratory misdiagnosis by UHB histopathologists of specimens from NBT patients, despite there having been assurances by UHB that the problems had been overcome' and 'UHB continued to refuse to allow slides to be looked at by NBT histopathologists.' Dr Morse, then NBT medical director, said that unless an external review was arranged, he would report the matter to the Healthcare Commission. In August 2008, Graham Rich gave a written assurance that an external review had been requested. It never happened. The Royal College of Pathologists was contacted but claims it never received the formal agreement of both trusts to do the review. And without an invitation, the royal college is powerless to intervene even if serious misdiagnosis is occurring.

Forced into action by the *Eye*, UHB has organised its own external review using a private company called Medical Solutions, which already does the trust's breast cancer receptor testing, and so has a financial stake in one of the four areas of concern. Hardly independent. 3,500 slides across the entire pathology service are going to be chosen at random for one year (2007) to see if there is a significant error rate. If UHB had proper prospective audit, it would already know what it's error rate is for subspecialties and pathologists. The random selection will not include any errors prior to 2007 and, according to one statistician, 'is fraught with methodological problems and extremely unlikely to get to the heart of the problem.'

Specialist pathology is not simply making a diagnosis of, say, benign or malignant but recognising other features of the tissue that should guide very complex treatment in discussion with the entire team. There is a national shortage of specialist pathologists, and Bristol can only provide a safe service by merging the expertise of its two trusts. As one senior consultant at NHS Bristol put it: 'We've been trying to do this ever since I arrived in Bristol 25 years ago.' The external review is looking for the wrong problem in the wrong place. It's changing the culture and service afterwards that matters. Time to grow up and get on with it.

BLOWING YOUR OWN WHISTLE:
WISE UP AND SPEAK UP

The NHS needs more people speaking up from the bottom and fewer shouting out from the top. The secret of speaking up, whether you're a health service worker or user, is to try to work as a team and intervene early, before a potential problem becomes a definite disaster. And try to give appropriate praise and positive feedback too (something that the British aren't terribly good at).

Americans seem to find feedback much easier, and their Joint Commission (like our Care Quality Commission but with bigger balls) has even launched it's own Speak Up campaign (reproduced, slightly adapted, below). If you want access to the same factual knowledge your doctor has, I'd recommend the NHS Clinical Knowledge Summaries (www.cks.library.nhs.uk/home). If you want to share other people's experiences of health and illness, try Health Talk Online (www.healthtalkonline.org). If you want to share your own experience of the service or treatment with others, or check it out first, there's www.patientopinion.org.uk and www.iwantgreatcare.org. But the best feedback of all is to look the person who's treating you in the eye and tell them directly, trying to be constructive but not skirting around the issues. You are a Vice President of the Royal College of Patients, after all.

SPEAK UP QUESTIONS
ADAPTED SLIGHTLY FROM THE JOINT COMMISSION
www.jointcommission.org

Speak up if you have questions or concerns. If you still don't understand, ask again. It's your body and you have a right to know.

- Your health is very important. Do not worry about being embarrassed if you don't understand something that your doctor, nurse or other healthcare professional tells you. If you don't understand because you speak another language, ask for someone who speaks your language. You have the right to get free help from someone who speaks your language.
- Don't be afraid to ask about safety. If you're having surgery, ask the doctor to mark the area that is to be operated on.
- Don't be afraid to tell the nurse or the doctor if you think you are about to get the wrong medicine.
- Don't be afraid to tell a healthcare professional if you think he or she has confused you with another patient.

Pay attention to the care you get. Always make sure you're getting the right treatments and medicines by the right healthcare professionals. Don't assume anything.

- Tell your nurse or doctor if something doesn't seem right.
- Expect healthcare workers to introduce themselves. Look for their identification (ID) badges. A new mother should know the person she hands her baby to. If you don't know who the person is, ask for their ID.
- Notice whether your caregivers have washed their hands.

Hand washing is the most important way to prevent infections. Don't be afraid to remind a doctor or nurse to do this.

- Know what time of the day you normally get medicine. If you don't get it, tell your nurse or doctor.
- Make sure your nurse or doctor checks your ID. Make sure he or she checks your wristband and asks your name before he or she gives you your medicine or treatment.

Educate yourself about your illness. Learn about the medical tests you get, and your treatment plan.

- Ask your doctor about the special training and experience that qualifies him or her to treat your illness.
- Look for information about your condition. Good places to get that information are from your doctor, your library, respected websites and support groups.
- Write down important facts your doctor tells you. Ask your doctor if he or she has any written information you can keep.
- Read all medical forms and make sure you understand them before you sign anything. If you don't understand, ask your doctor or nurse to explain them.
- Make sure you know how to work any equipment that is being used in your care. If you use oxygen at home, do not smoke or let anyone smoke near you.

Ask a trusted family member or friend to be your advocate (adviser or supporter).

- Your advocate can ask questions that you may not think about when you are stressed.
- Ask this person to stay with you, even overnight, when you are hospitalised. You will be able to rest better. Your advocate can help make sure you get the right medicines and treatments.

- Your advocate can also help remember answers to questions you have asked. He or she can speak up for you when you cannot speak up for yourself.
- Make sure this person understands the kind of care you want. Make sure he or she knows what you want done about life support and other life-saving efforts if you are unconscious and not likely to get better.
- Go over the consents for treatment with your advocate before you sign them. Make sure you both understand exactly what you are about to agree to.
- Make sure your advocate understands the type of care you will need when you get home. Your advocate should know what to look for if your condition is getting worse. He or she should also know whom to call for help.

Know what medicines you take and why you take them. Medicine errors are the most common healthcare mistakes.

- Ask about why you should take the medication. Ask for written information about it, including its brand and generic names. Also ask about the side effects of all medicines.
- If you do not recognise a medicine, double-check that it is for you. Ask about medicines that you are to take by mouth before you swallow them. Read the contents of the bags of intravenous (IV) fluids. If you're not well enough to do this, ask your advocate to do it.
- If you are given an IV, ask the nurse how long it should take for the liquid to run out. Tell the nurse if it doesn't seem to be dripping right (too fast or too slow).
- Whenever you get a new medicine, tell your doctors and nurses about allergies you have, or negative reactions you have had to other medicines.
- If you are taking a lot of medicines, be sure to ask your doctor or pharmacist if it is safe to take those medicines

together. Do the same thing with vitamins, herbs and over-the-counter drugs.

- Make sure you can read the handwriting on prescriptions written by your doctor. If you can't read it, the pharmacist may not be able to either. Ask somebody at the doctor's office to print the prescription, if necessary.
- Carry an up-to-date list of the medicines you are taking in your purse or wallet. Write down how much you take and when you take it. Go over the list with your doctor and other caregivers.

Use a hospital, clinic, surgery centre, or other type of healthcare organisation that has been carefully checked out. For example, the Healthcare Commission (now part of the Care Quality Commission) visits hospitals to see if they are meeting quality standards. Ask to see the latest inspection report.

- Ask about the healthcare organisation's experience in taking care of people with your type of illness. How often do they perform the procedure you need? What special care do they provide to help patients get well?
- If you have more than one hospital to choose from, ask your doctor which one has the best care for your condition.
- Before you leave the hospital or other facility, ask about follow-up care and make sure that you understand all of the instructions.
- Go to the Healthcare Commission at www.healthcarecommission.org.uk and read more about the patient safety and quality standards at all the hospitals or clinics you could choose from.

Participate in all decisions about your treatment. You are the centre of the healthcare team.

- You and your doctor should agree on exactly what will be done during each step of your care.
- Know who will be taking care of you. Know how long the treatment will last. Know how you should feel.
- Understand that more tests or medications may not always be better for you. Ask your doctor how a new test or medication will help.
- Keep copies of your medical records from previous hospital stays and share them with your healthcare team. This will give them better information about your health history.
- Don't be afraid to ask for a second opinion. If you are unsure about the best treatment for your illness, talk with one or two additional doctors. The more information you have about all the kinds of treatment available to you, the better you will feel about the decisions made.
- Ask to speak with others who have had the same treatment or operation you may have to have. They may help you prepare for the days and weeks ahead. They may be able to tell you what to expect and what worked best for them.
- Talk to your doctor and your family about your wishes regarding resuscitation and other life-saving actions.

FURTHER READING

Patient Safety by Charles Vincent (Churchill Livingstone) is a wise, balanced, insightful and motivating overview. I should have read it earlier.

Better and *Complications*, two books by American surgeon Atul Gawande (Profile), are gripping and humane accounts of the complexity, triumphs and challenges of healthcare. Gawande opts for understanding rather than exposure, and promotes positive deviancy rather than nihilistic ranting. I fear he may have a point.

How Shall I Tell the Dog? by Miles Kington (also Profile) is an object lesson in how to die with style and humour, and how to make death earn its living.

CUT OUT AND KEEP

THE ROYAL COLLEGE OF PATIENTS
Vice President

DR PHIL

Phil Hammond is a GP, writer, comic and broadcaster. He has worked in sexual health and as a lecturer in medical communication at two universities (Birmingham and Bristol). He currently works part-time as a GP and will continue until the GMC tells him to stop. Phil is still *Private Eye*'s medical correspondent and possibly the only comedian to have appeared at a Public Inquiry. He has been a regular panellist on *Have I Got News for You*, *The News Quiz*, *The Now Show* and *Countdown*, and presented five series of *Trust Me, I'm a Doctor* on BBC2. Dr Phil is a Patron of the Herpes Viruses Association and a Vice President of both the Patients' Association and the Royal College of Patients.

Phil is married and lives in Somerset with two of everything (kids, dogs, cats, ponies and testes). He also has two other books, *Medicine Balls* and *Why Does it Hurt When I Pee?*